PRACTICAL PAEDIATRIC PRESCRIBING

PRACTICAL PAEDIATRIC PRESCRIBING

HOW TO PRESCRIBE THE MOST COMMON DRUGS

Will Carroll BM BCh, MA, MD, FRCPCH
Consultant Paediatrician and Honorary Reader in Child Health, Staffordhire Children's Hospital at Royal Stoke and Keele University,
Stoke-on-Trent, UK

Francis Gilchrist MB ChB, FRPCH, PhD
Senior Lecturer, Institute of Science and Technology in Medicine, Keele University,
Keele, UK
Paediatric Respiratory Consultant, Staffordshire Children's Hospital at Royal Stoke,
Stoke on Trent, UK

Michael Mitchell MPharm, MSc ClinPharm
Clinical Pharmacist, Paediatric & Neonatal Intensive Care Unit, Royal Hospital for Children,
Glasgow, UK

Helen Sammons MB ChB, MRCPCH, MD
Consultant Paediatrician, North Devon District Hospital, Raleigh Heights,
Barnstaple, UK
Honarary Associate Professor of Child Health, University of Nottingham,
Nottingham, UK

Jyothi Srinivas MBBS, FRCPCH, PG Dip (Med Ed)
Consultant Paediatrician and Deputy DME, Milton Keynes University Hospital,
Milton Keynes, UK
Honorary Senior Clinical Lecturer, University Of Buckingham Medical School,
Buckingham, UK

For additional online content visit StudentConsult.com

ELSEVIER   London   New York   Oxford   Philadelphia   St Louis   Sydney   2021

PRACTICAL PAEDIATRIC PRESCRIBING   ISBN: 978-0-7020-7612-1

Notices

Practitioners and researchers must always rely on their own experience and knowledge in evaluating and using any information, methods, compounds or experiments described herein. Because of rapid advances in the medical sciences, in particular, independent verification of diagnoses and drug dosages should be made. To the fullest extent of the law, no responsibility is assumed by Elsevier, authors, editors or contributors for any injury and/or damage to persons or property as a matter of products liability, negligence or otherwise, or from any use or operation of any methods, products, instructions, or ideas contained in the material herein.

Senior Content Strategist: Pauline Graham
Content Strategist: Alexandra Mortimer
Content Development Specialist: Carole McMurray
Content Coordinator: Susan Jansons
Project Managers: Anne Collett and Joanna Souch
Design: Brian Salisbury
Marketing Manager: Deborah Watkins

Printed in Poland

Last digit is the print number: 9 8 7 6 5 4 3 2 1

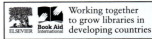

Contents

Contents

Preface

The journey for this small book began in 2012. At the time I was working in Derbyshire Children's Hospital, a centre in which I had the pleasure of working with two of my co-editors and that had a particular academic focus on paediatric pharmacology. With the help of our senior lecturer in paediatric pharmacology and a host of medical students I conducted a census of drug use on the children's wards. The hope was that I could identify a 'top 10' list of medicines for children that could be considered core knowledge for our undergraduate medical students.

After months of study, it became clear that close to 100 medicines were used fairly often on a general paediatric ward. I also quickly recognized that I did not know as much about how these medicines worked as I should. What turned into a small project to assist curriculum design turned into a series of four review articles for the most commonly prescribed drugs: paracetamol, ibuprofen, salbutamol and codeine. Despite more than 10 years of experience as a consultant paediatrician I found that each of these articles changed how I used these medicines in practice. My better understanding led to improvements in patient care.

I also found a helpful and memorable structure for concisely summarizing the important properties of medicines relevant to paediatric practice and I began to make my own notes. In each 'chapter' of this book we consider the 'ABCDE' of the relevant drug(s). Where possible, we have used original research studies to provide data on what is known about **A**bsorption, **B**iological effects, **C**learance, **D**osing and side **E**ffects in children. When data on different age groups are available, we have attempted to summarize these.

Whilst this book is not intended to replace existing formularies for prescribing purposes, it adds far more detail about how each medicine works. In turn, we hope this knowledge will assist students and clinicians to use the medicines available better in individual children.

It is also *interesting*!

We were amazed to discover that humble lactulose is, in fact, a prebiotic. I now understand why oral paracetamol is relatively ineffective in children with immediate postoperative pain. The tissue distribution of macrolides is fascinating. In fact, I think that there is at least one really interesting fact about each medicine covered in this book. I hope you agree. Uncovering these gems of knowledge has been a true team effort. This book would not have been possible without the tremendous work done by each chapter author and my knowledgeable editorial team.

We hope that you will use this book as you encounter children in your clinical practice. Each chapter is intended to be short enough to read 'on the go' and is aimed at students, trainees and more experienced clinicians. We hope it will also allow you to discover and share some of the editors' love of pharmacology.

Will Carroll

Acknowledgements

The editors would like to acknowledge three inspirational clinicians who stimulated our interest in medicines: Professor Imti Choonara, Dr Sharon Conroy and Professor Warren Lenney. All the editors would like to thank their partners and children for their support. Each chapter stole time from weekends and holidays that we can never wholly repay. Thank you.

List of Contributors

Nabeel Abdul-Kareem MBBS, MD, MRCPCH

Speciality Registrar, Peninsula Rotation
Carbamazepine
Ethosuximide
Levetiracetam
Midazolam
Sodium valproate

Imran Ali MBBS, BSc

Academic Foundation Doctor
Staffordshire Children's Hospital at Royal
Stoke
Furosemide

Lateefat Arije MBBS, MPH, MRCPCH

Milton Keynes University Hospital
Clarithromycin

Rhiannon Austin

Clinical Research Fellow, University
of Liverpool
Aminophylline and theophylline
Beclometasone dipropionate
Magnesium

Amal Azher Anwer BSc, MSc

Keele Medical School
Omalizumab

Johanna Baker MB ChB, MRCPCh

Wexham Park Hospital
Salbutamol

Christopher Bakewell MB BCh, BSc, MRCPCH

Milton Keynes University Hospital and
Thames Valley Paediatric Deanery
Montelukast

Sarah Band MB ChB, MRCPCH, DTM&H

Paediatric ST3
Royal Stoke University Hospital,
University Hospital of North Midlands
Metronidazole

Maxim John Levy Barnett MB ChB

Milton Keynes University Hospital
Clarithromycin

Supriyo Basu MBBS, DCH, MRCPCH

Consultant
Paediatric Endocrinology & Diabetes
Oxford University Hospitals NHS
Foundation Trust
Azithromycin

Reethee Bhatt MB ChB

John Radcliffe Children's Hospital,
Oxford;
Milton Keynes University Hospital Trust
Hydrocortisone

James Chapman MBBS, FRCPCH

Consultant Paediatrician, Staffordshire
Children's Hospital at Royal Stoke
Ketamine

Justin Collis MB ChB, BA

University of Buckingham
Mannitol

Jenny Cooper MB ChB, MRCPCH

Oxford University Hospitals NHS
Foundation Trust
Omeprazole

Samuel Crocker MB ChB, MRCPCH

North Devon District Hospital
Desmopressin
Insulin
Levothyroxine sodium
Oxybutynin hydrochloride

Rebecca Duncombe MBBS, MRCPCH, PgCert

Paediatric Consultant, Buckinghamshire NHS Trust
Ibuprofen

Sheila Farnan MB ChB, MRCPCH

Specialist Registrar, North Devon District Hospital, Peninsular Rotation
Gaviscon®
Lactulose
Senna

Amruta Amit Fulmali MBBS, MRCPCH, MRCPI

Torbay and South Devon NHS Foundation Trust, Torquay
Cefuroxime
Fluticasone
Gentamicin

Akshat Goel MBBS, MD, DNB

Paediatric MTI Fellow in Royal Stoke University Hospital, UHNM, Stoke-on-Trent
Isoniazid

Ellen Grose-Hodge MMedEd

Keele University/Keele University School of Medicine
Second-generation antihistamines
Chloral hydrate
Tranexamic acid

Dan Hawcutt BSc, MB ChB, MD, MRCPCH

Senior Lecturer Paediatric Clinical Pharmacology, Women's and Children's Health
University of Liverpool
Aminophylline and theophylline
Heparin (unfractionated)
Hydrocortisone
Ibuprofen
Low-molecular-weight heparin (LMWH)
Methotrexate
Methyprednisolone
Prednisolone

Alihussein Jaffer MPharm

Clinical Pharmacist, Milton Keynes University Hospital
Meropenem
Piperacillin with tazobactam (Tazocin®)

Yasmin Jaffer MBBS, DMCC, PGCert (Med Ed)

ST2 Paediatric Doctor
Children's Hospital, John Radcliffe, Oxford
Ipratropium bromide

Bridget Margaret Hope Kemball MPhil

Medical Student, Keele University
Colomycin
Dornase alfa (DNAse)

Sheethal Kodagali MBBS, MRCPCH, DNB

Department of Paediatrics, John Radcliffe Hospital, Oxford University NHS Foundation Trust, Oxford
Calcium

Mithilesh Lal MD, MRCP, FRCPCH

Consultant Neonatologist, Clinical
Director for Neonatal services
Associate Medical Director
(Revalidation),The James Cook University
Hospital, South Tees Foundation NHS
Trust
Dobutamine
Dopamine
Surfactant: pulmonary

Richard Lin MB ChB, BSc

Milton Keynes University Hospital,
Buckinghamshire Healthcare Trust,
Oxford Foundation School
Amoxicillin

Emma Lovell MBBS

North Devon District Hospital
Codeine phosphate
Morphine

**Heather McNeilly BA, Hons, MBBS,
MRCPCH, PGCert MedEd, FHEA**

Clinical Education Fellow
George Eliot Hospital NHS Foundation
Trust
Paraldehyde

**Francesca Mitchell MBBS, BSc,
MRCPCH**

Milton Keynes University Hospital
Dexamethasone

**James Moss MB ChB, MPharm,
PGDip, MRCPCH**

Alder Hey Children's NHS Foundation
Trust, Liverpool
Department of Women's and Children's
Health, University of Liverpool, Liverpool
Heparin (unfractionated)
Low-molecular-weight heparin (LMWH)

Hiba Muhialdin MBBS

Junior Trust Doctor, E24 Paediatrics at
Milton Keynes University Hospital (MKUH)
Vitamin K (Phytomenadione)

**David Nwokeocha MB ChB, DCH,
MRCPCH**

Paediatric Registrar
Royal Stoke University Hospital, UHNM,
Stoke-on-Trent
Hyoscine hydrobromide

**Roy Osgood BMBS, BSc (Hons),
MRCPCH**

Oxford University Hospitals NHS Trust
Ondansetron

Tejaswi Patel BMBS

Nottingham
Trimethoprim

Dorothea Paul MD

Paediatric ED ST1 Clinical Fellow
St Mary's Hospital, Imperial College NHS
University Trust, London
Vitamin D

**Arumuga Prabhu Rajendran DCH,
MRCPCH, PG Cert**

Paediatric Gastroenterology Consultant
Paediatrician, Luton and Dunstable
University Hospital
Ciclosporin
Phosphate (enema and supplements)

**Sajida Rasul MB ChB, BSc, MRCPCH
MSc**

Clinical Research Facility, Alder Hey
Children's Hospital NHS Trust and The
University of Liverpool
Hydrocortisone
Ibuprofen
Methotrexate
Methyprednisolone
Prednisolone

Ghulam Raza MBBS, DCH, MRCPI Paediatrics, MRCPCH

Specialty Trainee Paediatrics
HEE South West – Peninsula
Baclofen
Chloral hydrate

Lyndsey Rowley MB ChB, MRCPCH

Milton Keynes University Hospital NHS Trust
Acetylcysteine

Bethany Jane Seale MPhil

Keele University
Amitriptyline
Methylphenidate (Ritalin®, Medikinet®, Concerta XL®, Equasym XL®)

Krishna Shetye DCH, DNB, MRCPCH

Specialty Doctor Paediatrics, Milton Keynes University Hospital
Adrenaline (epinephrine)
Atropine

Rachel Smith MB ChB, MRCPCH

Royal Derby Hospital
Iron (ferrous sulfate, ferrous fumarate, sodium feredetate)
Sodium picosulphate

James Walker MPhil

Year 5 Medical Student
Royal Stoke University Hospital, UHNM, Stoke-on-Trent, Keele University
Abidec®
Ketamine
Warfarin

Hannah Walsh MB BCh, MRCPCH, DTMH

Paediatric Speciality Trainee, Peninsula Deanery
Ciprofloxacin
Erythromycin

Ben Walters

Year 5 Medical Student
Royal Stoke University Hospital, UHNM, Stoke-on-Trent
Atenolol
Melatonin

Chun Wai Wong MB ChB

Academic Foundation Year 2 Trainee
Royal Stoke University Hospital, UHNM, Stoke-on-Trent
Metronidazole

Jenny Wright BMBS

Academic Foundation Year Two Doctor
University Hospitals North Midlands Trust
Docusate
Domperidone
Lidocaine

Eleftheria Xilas BSc

Keele University
Ranitidine

Lefteris Zolotas MD, MSc, MRCPCH

University Hospitals of Derby and Burton NHS Foundation Trust
Amiloride
Captopril
Digoxin
Spironolactone

The Top Paediatric Drugs

Abidec®

CLINICAL PHARMACOLOGY

Why and when?	Abidec® is a **multivitamin** oral preparation for paediatric patients, given to *prevent* vitamin deficiencies and their respective impacts on health. Certain patient groups may be susceptible to developing vitamin deficiencies, such as children with malabsorption, and prophylaxis is often indicated in these groups. The need for additional vitamins varies by age and diet. In some countries, foods are supplemented with vitamins. In the UK the Department of Health recommends that **all children aged 6 months to 5 years are given supplements** containing vitamins A, C and D every day but only a small proportion of families are entitled to receive these on prescription.
Absorption	Abidec is absorbed from different parts of the gastrointestinal tract, as it contains multiple fat-soluble (A and D) and water-soluble (B group and C) vitamins. **Vitamin B** is **absorbed widely** and some is likely to be absorbed from the stomach because following gastrectomy vitamin B deficiencies are more common. **Vitamin A and D** are absorbed principally in the **duodenum with dietary fat**, whereas **vitamin C** is absorbed in the **jejunum and ileum**.
Biology	Abidec contains vitamins A, B_1, B_2, B_3, B_6, C and D. These have a wide range of physiological effects. Some catalyse biochemical processes and others act as hormones controlling endocrine axes. **Vitamin A** (retinol) is vital in retinal light transduction, allowing the perception of **vision**. It plays an important role in bone development, regulating the immune system and haematopoiesis. Severe deficiency leads to night blindness, follicular hyperkeratosis, poor growth and xerophthalmia. Even mild, subclinical deficiency impairs immune response and results in increased childhood mortality from infections. **Vitamin B_1** (thiamine) is a cardio- and neuro-protective **antioxidant**. It has a complicated mechanism of action involving the modulation of cellular glucose metabolism. Severe **deficiency** results in **beri-beri**, with polyneuropathy, muscle tenderness, heart failure and ophthalmoplegia. Vitamin B_2 (riboflavin) and B_3 (nicotinamide) play key roles in cellular aerobic respiration. Deficiency of vitamin B_2 leads to anaemia, mucositis, anorexia and nasolabial seborrhoea. Whilst some vitamin B_3 can be synthesized from tryptophan endogenously, deficiency leads to photosensitivity, dermatitis, diarrhoea and dementia (pellagra). **Vitamin B_6 (pyridoxine)** is a co-factor in neurotransmitter synthesis, amino acid and carbohydrate metabolism. Deficiency leads to **seizures**, hyperacusis, microcytic anaemia and neuropathy. Vitamin C (ascorbic acid) is an antioxidant, mitigating inflammatory actions of free radicals in different tissues. It is required for collagen and glycosaminoglycan synthesis, and deficiency causes scurvy, which results in poor wound healing, irritability, bruising, bleeding gums and aching bones. **Vitamin D** (cholecalciferol) is a fat-soluble vitamin. Under most circumstances 90% is produced in the skin via UV biosynthesis of skin sterols, but dietary vitamin D is absorbed in the duodenum. Vitamin D is converted to its biologically **active form** via **hydroxylation** in the **liver and the kidney**. It plays a pivotal role in maintaining bone health, and **deficiency** leads to **rickets** (osteomalacia and impaired growth). It also aids immune function.

PRACTICAL PRESCRIBING

Clearance	In general terms it is helpful to consider **water-soluble** and **fat-soluble** vitamins separately. Water-soluble vitamins readily dissolve in water and are absorbed into the tissues for immediate use. With the exception of vitamin B_6 (pyridoxine), which is stored and metabolized in the liver, they are excreted by the kidney and following dosing. Vitamins B_1, B_6 and C have a relatively long biological half-life of between 10 and 20 days in adults. However, the **body stores of water-soluble vitamins are more rapidly depleted during periods of starvation**. Young women with hyperemesis of pregnancy are at risk of water-soluble vitamin deficiency and require vitamin supplementation (particularly with vitamin B_1 (thiamine)) and if untreated they are at risk of **Wernicke encephalopathy**. **Fat-soluble vitamins** have a much **longer effective biological half-life**. As these are stored in body fat it is difficult to determine their half-life using conventional pharmacokinetic studies but estimates suggest that for vitamin A and D these are between **60 and 300 days**.
Dosing	Each 0.6 mL dose of Abidec contains: 1333 IU vitamin A (retinol), 0.4 mg vitamin B_1 (thiamine), 0.8 mg vitamin B_2 (riboflavin), 8 mg vitamin B_3 (nicotinamide), 0.8 mg vitamin B_6 (pyridoxine), 40 mg vitamin C (ascorbic acid) and 400 IU vitamin D (ergocalciferol). It is recommended that preterm neonates and children aged 1–17 years receive 0.6 mL daily. Children aged 1–11 months should be given 0.3 mL daily. For most age groups this dose gives a child roughly their daily requirement of each component vitamin (the recommended daily amount). It is used to *prevent* deficiency.
Administration	Abidec is administered by mouth via **oral drops**.
Side effects and interactions	Adverse effects are not expected from this medication as the constituent vitamins are a part of a healthy diet. The doses given are **far below those which would lead to toxicity**, there is a very large therapeutic window. Patients with peanut and soya allergies should not take this medication as **peanut oil is an ingredient** (an alternative, Dalivit®, does not but contains proportionally more vitamin A). Abidec should not be given to patients already receiving supplementation for vitamins the medication contains; this includes medicines such as alfacalcidol. Formula-fed infants should remain at 0.3 mL doses as infant formula is supplemented with vitamin D.
Monitoring	There is no extra monitoring required for patients taking Abidec; clinicians should be aware of symptoms of toxicity (such as drowsiness, vomiting and diarrhoea in hypervitaminosis A).
Cost	Abidec is fairly **cheap**. One 25 mL bottle of Abidec costs £3.68.

Acetazolamide

CLINICAL PHARMACOLOGY

Why and when?	Acetazolamide is a non-antimicrobial sulfonamide which is a non-competitive, reversible **inhibitor of carbonic anhydrase**. It is most commonly used in children to treat raised intracranial pressure in individuals with **idiopathic intracranial hypertension (IIH)** as it reduces the production of cerebrospinal fluid (CSF). Whilst there is no consensus and uncertainty remains about the use of acetazolamide for this indication, dosing recommendations are given in the British National Formulary for Children (BNFc) and the 2018 UK consensus statement on management of IIH.
	In the eye, it **decreases aqueous humour formation** so can be used to treat primary and secondary glaucoma. In the brain, acetazolamide also reduces excessive neuronal discharges so can be used as an antiepileptic, especially for absences. In the kidneys, it is a mild diuretic so can be used to treat fluid retention, although it is rarely used for this indication in children. In adults, acetazolamide can be used to prevent and treat **altitude sickness**.
Absorption and distribution	Acetazolamide is absorbed fairly efficiently from the gastrointestinal tract with the peak serum concentration being achieved after 2 hours; however, accurate data on absolute oral bioavailability are lacking in humans. Whilst pharmacodynamic data are sparse, it certainly has an action on the central nervous system (CNS) affecting both CSF production and neuronal function, therefore is **likely to cross the blood–brain barrier**. It is distributed throughout all body tissues. It can accumulate in tissues containing carbonic anhydrase such as the kidneys and red blood cells.
Biology	The actions of acetazolamide result from the inhibition of carbonic anhydrase. It acts **directly on the choroid plexus** to reduce CSF production. In the kidneys carbonic anhydrase converts carbon dioxide and water to hydrogen and bicarbonate. Acetazolamide inhibits this enzymatic reaction, resulting in decreased hydrogen ions in the renal tubules, which **increases the excretion of bicarbonate, sodium, potassium and water**. In the eye, carbonic anhydrase is involved in the production of aqueous humour through control of the cellular sodium pump. Acetazolamide **decreases aqueous humour formation** and lowers intraocular pressure. In the brain, acetazolamide inhibits CNS carbonic anhydrase, which increases intracellular CO_2, decreases intracellular pH and supresses any excessive neuronal discharge. Partial tolerance may develop to its antiepileptic activity.
Clearance	Acetazolamide is excreted unchanged in the urine. Renal clearance is enhanced in alkaline urine and the usual elimination **half-life is about 4 hours**. Clearance is reduced in individuals with renal impairment.

PRACTICAL PRESCRIBING

Dosing and administration	Acetazolamide is **usually administered orally** as immediate-release tablets (Diamox®) or sustained-release capsules (Diamox® SR). Intravenous preparations are available but intramuscular administration should be avoided as it is painful due to the solution being alkaline.
	For the treatment of glaucoma in children <12 years, the dose is **5 mg/kg 2–4 times daily** (maximum dose 750 mg daily). In children >12 years, the dose is **250 mg 3 times daily**. For glaucoma modified-release preparations are used.
	For the treatment of epilepsy the dose starts at **2.5 mg/kg 2–3 times daily** and can be increased to **5–7 mg/kg 2–3 times daily** (maximum dose 750 mg daily).
	When used to treat raised intracranial pressure (IIH) the dose is typically higher. Initial doses for children <11 years are **8 mg/kg 3 times a day**, increased if necessary **up to 100 mg/kg daily**. In adults the maximum dose used in research studies is 4 g daily with side effects being common at mean daily doses of 1.5 g. A popular starting dose of acetazolamide is 250–500 mg twice a day, with the majority of clinicians titrating the daily dose up.
Side effects and interactions	At higher doses, **side effects are very common**. Nearly all patients taking acetazolamide for intracranial hypertension suffer side effects, tingling of the fingers and toes being the most common.
	Long-term use of acetazolamide can lead to metabolic acidosis due to increased bicarbonate excretion sometimes exacerbated by elevated plasma chloride concentrations. Reduced citrate excretion with no effect on calcium excretion increases the risk of renal calculi. Acetazolamide can potentiate the effects of folic acid antagonists. It should not be given if the patient is known to be allergic to sulfonamides. Patients should be warned of the adverse side effects of acetazolamide that are well recognized and include increased risk of diarrhoea, fatigue, nausea, paraesthesia, tinnitus, vomiting, depression and, rarely, renal stones.
Monitoring	Routine drug concentration monitoring is not necessary. Electrolyte abnormalities are common with prolonged use and **serum electrolytes should be checked regularly** whilst establishing a maintenance dose and periodically thereafter.
Cost	Acetazolamide is **fairly cheap**. Oral acetazolamide costs approximately £0.45/g. Therefore even at the maximum dose (4 g/day) it will cost c.£700 per year of treatment.

Acetylcysteine

CLINICAL PHARMACOLOGY

Why and when?	Acetylcysteine (also known as N-acetylcysteine, NAC or Parvolex®) is most commonly used in the UK for treatment of **paracetamol overdose**. It is used in the intravenous (IV) form and is given in patients whose paracetamol level is above the treatment line on the paracetamol overdose treatment graph. Acetylcysteine should also be given immediately in any patient who presents more than 8 hours after overdose with paracetamol (until levels are available) or where the overdose has been staggered with a total of more than 150 mg/kg over a 24-hour period. Less commonly, the oral form of the drug can be used in neonates for **meconium ileus** or children with cystic fibrosis for the treatment of **distal intestinal obstruction syndrome**. Other uses include as an **ocular lubricant** in eye-drop form and as a **mucolytic** in children with tenacious bronchial secretions (oral or nebulized).
Absorption	Whilst it is most commonly used intravenously, acetylcysteine is **absorbed rapidly** after oral administration, with peak levels between 30 minutes and 1 hour after administration.
Biology	In paracetamol overdose, acetylcysteine is thought to act via a variety of mechanisms. Paracetamol and its **toxic metabolites** are converted to non-toxic forms both by **conjugation with sulfate and by conjugation with glutathione** in the liver. In overdose the demand for glutathione is higher than its regeneration, leaving paracetamol in its toxic form, which has the potential to cause hepatocellular damage. Acetylcysteine works by acting as a **glutathione surrogate**, being metabolized itself to glutathione and by increasing conjugation of the paracetamol with sulfate. This results in conversion of paracetamol and its metabolites to non-toxic forms **reducing the hepatotoxic effects of overdose**. Acetylcysteine is also thought to reduce the inflammatory response, which can contribute to hepatic necrosis. Acetylcysteine acts as a mucolytic through its free sulfhydryl group, which opens up the disulfide bonds present in mucus, therefore **lowering mucus viscosity and elasticity**. By this mechanism acetylcysteine can loosen respiratory secretions and treat meconium ileus and distal intestinal obstruction syndrome. By reducing the viscosity of ocular mucus, acetylcysteine acts as an ocular lubricant.
Clearance	The plasma **half-life is 2.5 hours** with no acetylcysteine detectable 10–12 hours after administration. Acetylcysteine undergoes extensive first-pass metabolism by cells of the small intestine (when taken orally) and the liver. Only a very small percentage of intact acetylcysteine molecules reach the tissues. Acetylcysteine is metabolized to form cysteine and disulfides. Cysteine is further metabolized to form glutathione and other metabolites. A proportion (up to 38%) of acetylcysteine is excreted unchanged in the urine following IV dosing.

PRACTICAL PRESCRIBING

Dosing	The IV dosing regimen for treatment of paracetamol overdose in all ages, including neonates, is initially 150 mg/kg over 1 hour (loading dose), followed by 50 mg/kg over 4 hours (12.5 mg/kg/h) and finally 100 mg/kg over 16 hours (6.25 mg/kg/h). **When calculating the dose of IV acetylcysteine the child's actual weight should be used, up to a maximum of 110 kg**.
Administration	The solution for injection when being used intravenously is preferably made up with 5% glucose but 0.9% sodium chloride solution may be used as an alternative if needed. The IV dosing for paracetamol overdose is given as **three consecutive IV infusions across a total of 21 hours**. This may sometimes need to be extended further depending on clinical situations or if blood results remain abnormal.
	Orally, acetylcysteine comes as granules, or the injection solution can be diluted to a concentration of 50 mg/mL and taken orally. Acetylcysteine has a bitter taste so fruit juice or cola drink may be used as the diluent to make it more palatable. In rare cases where IV access is not possible, acetylcysteine can be given orally for paracetamol overdose, although it is not licensed in this form in the UK.
Drug errors and safety	Relatively high doses of acetylcysteine, up to 500 mg/kg, can be given without any toxic effects being seen. Clinically significant **anaphylactoid reactions** to IV acetylcysteine are reported in **around 10%** of patients in retrospective studies. The actual rates may be higher as prospective studies tend to show higher rates of reactions. Reactions usually occur during or soon after the first infusion and when **higher rates** of administration are used. Most are limited to cutaneous features (urticaria, pruritis and angioedema) but more severe systemic symptoms do occur. These reactions are more common in patients that have low or absent paracetamol levels or in children with a history of asthma. Treatment of any adverse effects is symptomatic. **A previous reaction** to acetylcysteine is **NOT a contraindication** to further courses of treatment; however, future treatments may need to be given at a **slower rate** and **prophylactic antihistamines** given prior to treatment.
Monitoring	Acetylcysteine can cause a slight rise in the international normalized ratio (INR) and prothrombin time, therefore these should be monitored before and at the end of the infusion regimen.
Cost	The solution for infusion intravenously comes in 10 mL vials each containing 2 g of acetylcysteine and costs between £21 and £25 for 10 ampoules. Oral acetylcysteine sachets containing 200 mg granules are more expensive at around £75 for 20 sachets.

Aciclovir

CLINICAL PHARMACOLOGY

Why and when?	Aciclovir is an **antiviral medication**. It is a safe and effective therapy for herpes simplex virus (HSV) infections. It is also used to treat chickenpox and shingles. Aciclovir is effective in patients with normal as well as deficient immune status. It is a synthetic, purine nucleoside analogue that has anti-herpes activity. It is more effective against HSV-1 and HSV-2 infection than varicella-zoster infections. It is available in topical, parenteral and oral formulations, including an oral suspension formulation for paediatric use. Topical therapy has little role in paediatric practice and should be avoided in favour of alternative modes of delivery. It should never be used as a topical therapy in neonates.
Absorption	The **bioavailability of oral formulations is modest** and **variable**, with only 15–30% of the oral formulation being absorbed. Bioavailability is typically lower in neonates and younger children. After topical application of 5% cream or eye ointment it **penetrates the superficial epidermis and cornea well**, achieving concentrations of up to 50 times than that seen in the superficial epidermis with oral aciclovir. However, when used to treat herpes labialis (cold sores) the infected cell type is located in the basal epidermis and the concentrations achieved here are much lower, typically 100–150 times lower than in superficial cells, which may explain the **limited efficacy of topical treatments**.
	There is widespread tissue distribution following systemic administration, and high concentrations of drug are achieved in the kidneys, lungs, liver, myocardium and skin vesicles. Cerebrospinal fluid concentrations are approximately 50% of plasma concentrations. Aciclovir crosses the placenta, and breast-milk concentrations are approximately 3 times that of plasma concentrations, although there are no data on efficacy of *in utero* therapy or impact of aciclovir therapy on nursing infants. Aciclovir therapy in a nursing mother is not a contraindication to breastfeeding.
Biology	The favourable safety profile of aciclovir derives from its **requirement for activation** to its active form via phosphorylation by a viral enzyme, **thymidine kinase**. Thus aciclovir can only be activated in cells already infected with HSV that express the viral TK enzyme. Aciclovir selectively inhibits the replication of HSV types 1 and 2 (HSV-1, HSV-2) and varicella-zoster virus (VZV). After intracellular uptake, it is converted to aciclovir monophosphate by virally encoded thymidine kinase. This step does not occur to any significant degree in uninfected cells and thereby lends specificity to the drug's activity.
Clearance	The main route of elimination is renal, and dosage adjustments are necessary for renal insufficiency. Haemodialysis also eliminates aciclovir. Aciclovir is primarily excreted unchanged in urine, both by glomerular filtration and tubular secretion. Its usual **plasma half-life is 2–3 hours**.

PRACTICAL PRESCRIBING

Dosing	For herpes simplex infection the oral dose is 100 mg 5 times a day for 5 days in children under 2 years of age and 200 mg 5 times a day for 5 days from 2 to 17 years of age. The dose is doubled for children who are immunocompromised or if the absorption is impaired. Aciclovir is given intravenously if central nervous system (CNS) infection is suspected or confirmed. Doses of 20 mg/kg given 8-hourly are recommended for neonates and babies up to 3 months. Older children aged 3 months–12 years should have 250 mg/m^2 8-hourly and children aged 12-17 years should have 5 mg/kg 8-hourly. Doses may be doubled and duration of treatment extended beyond 5 days in cases of VZV in the immunocompromised or where encephalitis is suspected. Dose modification is recommended for patients with reduced estimated GFR and in obese individuals. Topical preparations of 5% are available and can be applied to lesions every 4 hours, starting at the first sign of attack. The ointment also has to be applied 5 times a day and is more effective when started early. Topical therapy has modest effectiveness and has a limited role.
Administration	Oral liquid preparations are available in different flavours. **Oral aciclovir is a prescription-only drug**, which is available in a wide range of formulations and concentrations (200 mg/5 mL and 400 mg/5 mL). Dispersible tablets are available as 200 mg, 400 mg and 800 mg. **IV infusion is given slowly** over 1 hour after diluting with 0.9% sodium chloride solution and rapid infusions should be avoided.
Drug errors and safety	Aciclovir has an **exceptional safety profile**. Toxicity is observed typically only in rare circumstances, e.g. when high doses are given rapidly to a dehydrated child. High doses of aciclovir are associated with neurotoxicity and prolonged use can cause neutropenia. One uncommon but important complication of long-term use of aciclovir is the **selection for aciclovir-resistant HSV strains**, which usually occurs from **mutations in the HSV-TK gene**. Resistance is rarely observed in paediatric practice but should be considered in any patient who has been on long-term antiviral therapy and who has an HSV or VZV infection that fails to clinically respond to aciclovir therapy.
Monitoring	It is important to maintain adequate hydration for children who are on aciclovir. Monitoring is usually **dependent upon the underlying reason for treatment**. Children with suspected VZV or HSV encephalitis or congenital HSV/VZV infections are often very sick and require significant monitoring.
Cost	Aciclovir is **moderately expensive**. The cost of oral aciclovir (200 mg/5 mL) suspension is £35.47 per 125 mL bottle. Tablets are cheaper and dispersible tablets cost £2 for 25 200 mg tablets. IV preparations are expensive and cost around £40 per gram. IV aciclovir is available in 250 mg, 500 mg and 1 g vials.

Adrenaline (epinephrine)

CLINICAL PHARMACOLOGY

Why and when?	Adrenaline is a **sympathomimetic** drug and a potent stimulator of adrenergic receptors. This is particularly helpful in **anaphylaxis** where airway oedema, bronchospasm and hypotension all threaten life. **α-receptor** stimulation results in **vasoconstriction** tending to increase the blood pressure and reduce swelling, whereas **β-receptor** stimulation results in **bronchodilation** and **increased cardiac contractility and rate**. It is used as a bolus in **cardiac arrest**, as an infusion in the treatment of hypotension, to control bleeding or prolong local anaesthesia.
Absorption	Adrenaline is **not effective orally** because it is rapidly conjugated and oxidized in the gastrointestinal mucosa and liver. **Subcutaneous absorption is slow** because of local vasoconstriction but is more rapid after **IM injection** (onset of action **30–90 sec**, max effect at 4–10 min) and almost immediate when given **IV or IO** (onset **30 sec**, peak 3–5 min). When inhaled it works quickly, but mainly acts on respiratory tract; however, dose-dependent systemic effects occur.
Biology	1. Blood pressure – adrenaline is a **potent vasopressor**. It has three main effects: positive inotropic and positive chronotropic action on heart (β_1) and vasoconstriction (α). Low doses cause blood pressure to fall as vasodilator β_2-receptors are more sensitive than constrictor α-receptors. 2. Cardiac – adrenaline **increases cardiac output**. It acts on β_1-receptors of the myocardium, the cells of the pacemaker and conducting tissues. Heart rate increases, and cardiac systole is shorter. The work of the heart and its oxygen consumption are increased and cardiac efficiency is lessened. 3. Vascular effects – it markedly **reduces peripheral blood flow** due to **cutaneous vasoconstriction** (α) and **increased blood flow in skeletal muscles** via β_2-mediated vasodilation. 4. Respiratory effects – it is a **bronchodilator** (β_2) which also reduces bronchial secretions and congestion within the mucosa (α). It also inhibits mast cell secretion (β_2).

Effects of receptors	Receptors			
	α_1	α_2	β_1	β_2
	↑ Vasoconstriction ↑ Peripheral vascular resistance ↓ Mucosal oedema	↓ Insulin release ↓ Noradrenaline (norepinephrine) release	↑ Inotropy ↑ Chronotropy	↑ Bronchodilation ↑ Vasodilation ↑ Glycogenolysis ↓ Mediator release

Clearance	Adrenaline is **rapidly inactivated** in the liver and adrenergic neurons. It does not cross blood–brain barrier. Its plasma **half-life is 2–3 min**. It is excreted in urine mainly as inactive metabolites. If exposed to light or air, it turns pink from oxidation to adenochrome and then brown from formation of polymers. It is incompatible with bicarbonate and alkaline solutions.

PRACTICAL PRESCRIBING

Dosing	**The dose depends on indication**. It is available in 1 mg/mL (1 in 10,000) and 0.1 mg/mL (1 in 10000) concentrations and via auto-injector.
	Cardiopulmonary resuscitation – 0.01 mg/kg (0.1 mL/kg of 1 in 10,000), to be repeated every 3–5 min by IO/IV route. If no IV/IO access, endotracheal tube dose is 0.1 mg/kg (0.1 mL/kg of 1 in 1000).
	Acute hypotension – initially 0.1 microgram (mcg)/kg/min IV, adjusted according to response up to 1.5 mcg/kg/min.
	Anaphylaxis – 0.15–0.5 mg IM. Doses may be repeated, if necessary, at 5-min intervals according to blood pressure, pulse and respiratory function. 1 month–5 years: 0.15 mg (0.15 mL of 1:1000 adrenaline), 6–11 years: 0.3 mg, 12–17 years: 0.5 mg.
	Life-threatening croup – 400 mcg/kg (max dose 5 mg), repeated after 30 min if necessary.
Administration	For continuous IV infusion, dilute 1 in 1000 (1 mg/mL) adrenaline with glucose 5% or sodium chloride 0.9% and give through a central venous catheter. For nebulization in croup, adrenaline 1 in 1000 solution may be diluted with sterile sodium chloride 0.9% solution to a volume of 5 mL. This usually takes between 5 and 8 min to deliver completely.
Drug errors and safety	**IV adrenaline should be used with extreme care**. Bolus use is <u>**only recommended in cardiac arrest**</u>. Always use a central line if available. Extravasation is a risk when using peripheral veins. If extravasation occurs, stop infusion; gently aspirate extravasated solution (do NOT flush the line); remove needle/cannula; elevate extremity. Initiate phentolamine and apply dry warm compresses.
	Patients with allergies at higher risk of anaphylaxis and carers must be trained to use their auto-injector. Patients must check **the expiry date** of the auto-injectors and obtain replacements before expiry. Lacerations, bent and embedded needles are reported in children uncooperative during injection. To minimize risk, hold the child's leg firmly in place and limit movement prior to and during injection. The needle should remain in the thigh for the least amount of time as possible (≈3 secs).
Monitoring	Patients receiving adrenaline are usually unwell. Monitor heart rate, blood pressure, site of infusion for blanching/extravasation. **Continuous cardiac monitoring is required** during continuous infusion.
Cost	Adrenaline in 1:10,000-strength ampoules cost around £69.40 for a pack of 10, whereas 1:1000 strength is priced around £87.62 for a pack of 10 ampoules. **Auto-injectors are considerably more expensive** although vary by brand. Epipen (2 per pack) costs c.£90.

Amiloride

CLINICAL PHARMACOLOGY

Why and when?	Amiloride is a **potassium-sparing diuretic**. It is primarily used as an adjunct to thiazide or loop diuretics to treat heart failure and oedematous conditions such as nephrotic syndrome and ascites. Amiloride induces diuresis concurrently with potassium retention. Therefore, it is often used when potassium preservation is desirable. As a diuretic, it reduces the systemic blood pressure and it is used in the treatment of hypertension.
Absorption and distribution	Amiloride is absorbed from the gastrointestinal tract. Under usual circumstances about half is absorbed but absorption is **significantly reduced if taken with food** (by about 30%). Protein binding is minimal.
Biology	Amiloride exerts its action by **blocking** the **epithelial sodium channels** in the late distal convoluted tubule and collecting duct, which inhibits sodium reabsorption from the lumen. This effectively reduces intracellular sodium, **decreasing the function of Na^+/ K^+-ATPase, leading to potassium retention and decreased calcium, magnesium and hydrogen excretion.** The sodium uptake capacity in the late distal convoluted tubule and collecting duct is limited and therefore the diuretic and antihypertensive effects are generally considered weak.
Clearance	Amiloride is not metabolized by the liver. **Half-life is between 6 and 9 hours**. About 50% of amiloride is excreted unchanged by the kidneys, while around 40% is excreted in the faeces. Renal impairment prolongs the half-life of amiloride.
Dosing	The dose is dependent on the age of the child. The recommended dose is 100–200 micrograms/kg twice a day. Children older than 11 years receive 5–10 mg twice day. Maximum daily dose is 20 mg. In severe renal impairment its use should be avoided. No dose adjustment is necessary for hepatic impairment.

PRACTICAL PRESCRIBING

Administration	Amiloride is administered orally and is available as tablets and oral solution. Tablets are available as 5 mg and the oral solution in strength of 5 mg/5 mL and may contain propylene glycol as an excipient.
Side effects and interactions	Amiloride may cause **hyperkalaemia and postural hypotension**. It is known that amiloride itself can cause various mild side effects such as abdominal pain, nausea, anorexia and mild skin rash. The gastrointestinal side effects can be reduced by administration with meals but this will reduce absorption. Other side effects are more generally associated with its diuretic effect or the underlying diseases being treated such as constipation, diarrhoea, dyspepsia, dry mouth and gastrointestinal bleeding. Neurological side effects include headache, agitation, confusion, encephalopathy, tremor, paraesthesia, weakness, dizziness and insomnia. It is also associated with cough, dyspnoea and nasal congestion. Other side effects are malaise, arrhythmias, palpitations, arthralgia, muscle cramp, jaundice, pruritus, rash, alopecia, tinnitus, urinary disturbances, visual disturbance and raised intraocular pressure.
	The antihypertensive and potassium-sparing effect of amiloride may be enhanced when it is administered with medications that reduce systemic blood pressure and cause hyperkalaemia.
Monitoring	**Routine monitoring of electrolytes is advised** especially when it is administered in patients with renal impairment. **In hyperkalaemia amiloride should be discontinued**. As with all diuretics it is important to monitor hydration status and be vigilant for fluid overload. **Weighing children and comparing the measurements with their growth centile are very helpful**. A child who has rapidly gained weight is likely to be suffering from fluid overload and may need adjustment to their diuretic regimen.
Cost	As with many medicines for children, the oral solution is considerably more expensive than the tablet form. There are many manufacturers of the oral solution and a bottle of 150 mL costs around £37. A packet of 28 5 mg tablets has a drug tariff price of £3.99.

Aminophylline and theophylline

CLINICAL PHARMACOLOGY

Why and when?	Aminophylline and theophylline are **methylxanthines**. Aminophylline is a stable mixture of theophylline and ethylenediamine, which gives it greater solubility in water. They are used for severe and **life-threatening asthma** exacerbations and maintenance of **chronic severe asthma**, respectively. Use of theophylline in chronic asthma is only recommended when other interventions have not controlled symptoms. IV aminophylline is of no benefit in the mild–moderate asthma exacerbations. It is not routinely used in children <2 years; however, recent SIGN guidelines suggest it can be 'considered for children 12 months or older'. Aminophylline should not be used in children already taking theophylline.
Absorption	Theophylline is given orally in a modified-release preparation, and is well absorbed from the gastrointestinal (GI) tract. Aminophylline is given as a **slow IV bolus followed by a continuous infusion**. Once administered, **aminophylline is converted to theophylline**. Metabolism of theophylline is by hepatic cytochrome P450 enzymes. Oral theophylline reaches maximum plasma concentration within 2 hours. Its absorption has large interpatient variability and is affected by food intake and time taken.
Biology	Theophylline acts on **bronchial smooth muscle**. It inhibits phosphodiesterase isoenzymes which inactivate cyclic adenosine monophosphate (cAMP). This leads to an **increase in cAMP** and bronchodilation. Theophylline also has an adenosine receptor antagonistic effect likely to contribute to bronchodilation and a weak anti-inflammatory effect inhibiting synthesis of inflammatory mediators from mast cells and basophils.
	Theophylline, due to its wide distribution, has effects on many other systems. It is a *central nervous system* stimulant leading to heightened alertness and increased respiratory rate but also nervousness, tremor and sleep disruption. *Cardiovascularly*, it is a positive chronotrope and inotrope with smooth muscle vasodilation, which leads to an increase in heart rate and systemic vasodilation, but cerebral vasoconstriction. It has a weak diuretic effect on the *kidney*.
	In acute severe asthma, aminophylline has a worse risk:benefit ratio than β_2-adrenoceptor agonists. Its place in acute treatment is contested as IV magnesium sulfate may be safer and more efficacious.
Clearance	Theophylline is mainly cleared **hepatically by first-order kinetics** but becomes zero-order at high plasma levels. Less than 15% of administered theophylline is excreted unchanged in the urine. Aminophylline's **half-life has a wide variation** depending on age, genetic and environmental differences from **3.5–36 hours** (it is approximately 8 hours in a well adult).

PRACTICAL PRESCRIBING

Dosing	Aminophylline: for use in severe acute asthma management, a slow IV injection of 5 mg/kg (max 500 mg per dose) is given to those not on regular oral dosing. This is then followed by an IV infusion. The dose of the IV infusion is age- and weight-calculated. From 1 month to 11 years the infusion should be commenced at 1 mg/kg/h and for a child aged 12–17 years should be commenced at 500–700 micrograms/kg/h and rate adjusted as per theophylline-plasma concentration. **To avoid excessive dosage in obese patients the dose should be calculated on the basis of ideal weight for height**.

Oral theophylline: is available for use in chronic asthma via modified-release preparations. Whilst age-banded dosing is given, most children require approximately 9 mg/kg twice daily. It is necessary to adjust the dose based on theophylline-plasma level taken 4–6 hours after treatment at least 5 days after starting treatment. |
Administration	IV solution should be diluted with 5% glucose or 0.9% sodium chloride prior to administration. The oral forms are only available as tablets or capsules and the rate of absorption can vary between brands. **Therefore they should not be considered as interchangeable**.
Drug errors and safety	Due to the systemic effects, side effects and signs of toxicity include tachypnoea, tachycardia, arrhythmia and palpitation, tremor, headache, hyperthermia, nausea, hypokalaemia, seizures and hypotension. Nausea and vomiting are common side effects and should be treated with antiemetics. Dysrhythmia and seizure are the most worrying adverse effects and can be fatal. Therapeutic drug monitoring is required if treating a patient with aminophylline. **Serum concentrations >35 mg/L have been shown to have a greater risk of seizures and arrythmias.** Low albumin levels increase risk of toxicity and this should be kept in mind.
Monitoring	Therapeutic drug monitoring is required for patients treated with aminophylline and theophylline. Following an IV loading dose of aminophylline, the **plasma theophylline level should be in the range of 10–20 mg/L**. Further monitoring whilst on an IV infusion should be carried out if continuing for more than 24 hours. However, the current therapeutic range has been questioned in a recent systematic review, where outcomes did not improve in patients whose levels were between 10 mg/L and 20 mg/L in comparison to those with lower levels, and equally those patients with levels >20 mg/L were not found to have more adverse events than those with levels below 20 mg/L. A patient's clinical response and improvement should be also be used to guide therapy. Electrolytes should also be monitored along with plasma theophylline due to the increased risk of hypokalaemia with concurrent β_2-agonist use.
Cost	Aminophylline and theophylline are inexpensive. IV aminophylline 250 mg/10 mL solution costs £6.50 for 10 ampoules. Theophylline oral tablets/capsules range from £2.76 to £8.92 for 56 tablets.

Amitriptyline

CLINICAL PHARMACOLOGY

Why and when?

Amitriptyline is unlicensed in children; however, it is recommended for treatment of **neuropathic pain**. In adults it is also recommended for depressive illness and migraine prophylaxis. Neuropathic pain can be a part of many different diagnoses, including complex regional pain syndromes, autoimmune and degenerative neuropathies, and to counter the effects of cancer treatment.

Given the chronic nature of neuropathic pain and the lack of relief provided by routine analgesics, long-term neuromodulating agents, such as amitriptyline, have been increasingly prescribed.

Absorption

Amitriptyline **is almost completely but slowly absorbed** from the gastrointestinal tract after oral administration. Peak plasma concentrations are usually reached in 4–8 hours. Amitriptyline undergoes **first-pass metabolism** in the liver and its systemic bioavailability ranges from 33% to 62% after oral administration. Once it enters the systemic circulation it is extensively bound to plasma proteins (96%) but it passes easily into most tissues and **freely crosses the blood–brain barrier**.

Biology

Amitriptyline is a **tricyclic antidepressant**. It has several actions and its precise mechanism of action is unknown. It works in the central nervous system via the presynaptic blockade of noradrenaline and serotonin re-uptake pump. This **increases the number of neurotransmitters present in the synaptic cleft** and therefore increases neural transmission. It also exerts a lesser action by the presynaptic blockade of dopamine pump and the blockage of α-adrenergic receptors, muscarinic and histaminergic.

In animal studies (rats) amitriptyline **inhibits the blood–brain barrier** and **increases passage of other drugs**. It achieves this effect due to temporary inactivation of P-glycoprotein pumps. It is not yet known whether it has a similar effect in humans.

Clearance

Amitriptyline is metabolized by the cytochrome P450 system in the liver. Its primary metabolite is nortriptyline, which is another tricyclic antidepressant. Metabolites undergo glucuronidation or sulfonation prior to renal elimination. The typical **elimination half-life is relatively long at 25 hours**. This allows once-daily dosing in most instances. Most amitriptyline is excreted as metabolites in the urine.

PRACTICAL PRESCRIBING

Dosing	In children aged 2–11 years, a dose of 200–500 micrograms/kg once daily is recommended, with a maximum dose of 10 mg. For children aged 12–17 years, a starting dose of 10 mg once daily is recommended, with a maximum dose of 75 mg. It is advised that the dose is taken at night, due to the common side effect of drowsiness.
Administration	**Amitriptyline is given orally**. It can be given by an oral suspension or by tablets. It does not need to be given on an empty stomach but when once-daily dosing is attempted it is usually given at bedtime.
Drug errors and safety	Side effects of amitriptyline include urinary retention, visual disorders, dry mouth and dizziness. Older children should be advised amitriptyline can affect skilled tasks like driving and the effects of alcohol can be enhanced. There is risk of withdrawal when stopping amitriptyline and therefore the dose should be reduced gradually.

The oral suspension is available in three different concentrations, 10 mg/5 mL, 25 mg/5 mL and 50 mg/5 mL solutions. This is an important possible cause of error and care must be taken to stipulate both the dose and strength of any liquid forms. Parents must be warned if the strength is altered.

In overdose, amitriptyline is a dangerous cardiotoxic drug. It can cause intraventricular conduction delay leading to QRS prolongation. Overdose results in pupillary dilation, drowsiness and slow irregular respirations. It can also cause respiratory failure, hypotension and hypothermia. **Sodium bicarbonate is beneficial in overdose**. It has been shown to reverse QRS widening, hypotension and arrhythmias. |
| Monitoring | Children should be monitored for side effects. There is some limited evidence from adults that **side effects may reduce over time and can be minimized by starting at low doses before gradually increasing**. There is no routine monitoring for amitriptyline. |
| Cost | Amitriptyline is a relatively cheap medication in tablet form. It costs £0.65 for 28 × 25 mg tablets. Oral **suspension** is available as a special order form and is **much more expensive**. The 10 mg/mL solution is particularly expensive costing over £100 for 150 mL. Suspensions of 25 mg/mL and 50 mg/mL typically cost £18–20 for 150 mL. |

17

Amoxicillin

CLINICAL PHARMACOLOGY

Why and when?	Amoxicillin is a **broad-spectrum antibiotic**, indicated for children with **infections of the respiratory tract**, **ears**, skin and with *Helicobacter pylori*. It is commonly used in the treatment of **community-acquired pneumonia** in children, where it is as effective as IV antibiotics. It has specific indications for treatment of **listeria meningitis**, Lyme disease and anthrax.
	Amoxicillin is a very useful and widely used drug and is on the World Health Organization List of Essential Medicines. However, antimicrobial resistance is becoming more common. Amoxicillin has a **β-lactam ring**, and this is susceptible to damage or degradation by some strains of bacteria. Amoxicillin is sometimes given with clavulanic acid to increase antimicrobial activity against **β-lactamase-producing bacteria**. The combination of clavulanic acid with amoxicillin is **co-amoxiclav**. Care must be taken using **co-amoxiclav** to prevent the emergence of antimicrobial resistance.
Absorption	Amoxicillin is **rapidly and well absorbed via the oral route** and is stable against gastric mucosa. The oral bioavailability is 74–92%. For immediate-release formulation, peak concentration is reached within 1–2 hours. For extended-release formulation, peak concentration is reached in 3 hours. It has a somewhat larger volume of distribution in neonates and this is reflected in dosing guidelines.
Biology	Amoxicillin is an **aminopenicillin** that inhibits the cross-linking of peptidoglycans. It exerts this action by binding to intracellular penicillin-binding proteins, which are required to ensure the cross-linking of the external peptidoglycan cell wall occurs efficiently. This process **weakens the cell walls** of bacteria. The change in the osmotic gradient causes cell **swelling** and **lysis**, rendering amoxicillin **bactericidal**. The mechanism of action is shared with cephalosporins.
	Amoxicillin is a moderate spectrum antibiotic. It is effective against enterococci and Gram-negative aerobes, such as streptococci, *Haemophilus influenza*, *Proteus* sp., *E. coli*, *Shigella* and *Salmonella*. Amoxicillin also has activity against *Listeria monocytogenes* and *Borrelia*.
Clearance	In adults and older children the plasma half-life of amoxicillin is relatively short at about 1 hour. It is somewhat longer in neonates at around 3–4 hours. Amoxicillin is **renally excreted** with approximately 60% of oral intake excreted in the urine in the first 6–8 hours.

Non-allergic rash following amoxicillin

Up to 10% of children taking amoxicillin will develop a maculopapular rash >72 hours after starting a course. This is often misdiagnosed as an allergic reaction and yet this is rarely the case. It is unlikely to be a true allergic reaction and care must be taken before labelling a child as 'penicillin allergic'.

PRACTICAL PRESCRIBING

Dosing	The dose depends upon indication, age and in some instances weight but is the same for most indications except Lyme disease, Group B streptococcal infections, *Listeria* meningitis and *Helicobacter* eradication. In these situations expert advice should be taken and local guidelines consulted.

Neonates up to 7 days: **30 mg/kg** twice a day IV route only. Double dose in severe infection.

Neonates 7–28 days: **30 mg/kg** three times a day orally or IV. IV dose doubled in severe infection.

In children of **all ages over 28 days** the IV dose is 20-30 mg/kg three times a day (max 500 mg). This dose should be doubled in severe infection (max 1 g).

The oral doses are

Children 1–11 months: **125 mg** three times a day increased to 30 mg/kg in severe infection.

Children 1–4 years: **250 mg** three times a day increased in severe infection to 30 mg/kg 8-hourly.

Children 5–11 years: **500 mg** three times a day. Increase to 30 mg/kg (max 1 g) in severe infection.

Children 12–17 years: **500 mg** three times daily. Double dose in severe infection.

Administration	Amoxicillin is usually administered orally, available in solid and liquid formulations. The suspension is palatable and many children quite like the taste. Amoxicillin is available in peach, strawberry or lemon flavours for oral liquid formulations and sachets. For IV use it is necessary to dilute to a concentration of 50 mg/mL (100 mg/mL for neonates). The IV infusion should be given over 30 minutes when using doses above 30 mg/kg.
Drug errors and safety	Use of amoxicillin may increase the **risk of *C. difficile* infection**. Amoxicillin is contraindicated for a child **allergic to penicillin** or presenting with any hypersensitivity, such as **anaphylaxis**. Rashes are common but urticarial reactions suggest allergy and are an indication to stop or change treatment. Other adverse reactions include hypersensitivity angiitis, anxiety, confusion, dizziness, headache, insomnia, seizure, diarrhoea, **nausea**, **vomiting**, anaemia and cholestatic jaundice.
Monitoring	Routine drug monitoring is not required. Amoxicillin interacts with **warfarin**, **methotrexate** and anticoagulants. A child on anticoagulants should monitor International Normalized Ratio (INR) and adjust doses. Dose interval should be increased in children with renal impairment.
Cost	Amoxicillin is **cheap**. 100 mL of oral suspension (125 mg/5 mL or 250 mg/5 mL) costs £1–2. Amoxicillin tablets and capsules of 250 mg–500 mg cost between 2p and 5p each. 1 g of powder for injection costs around £2. Prescribing generic brands for amoxicillin saves costs. Co-amoxiclav preparations are only slightly more expensive (£1.50–6 for oral suspension).

Second-generation antihistamines

CLINICAL PHARMACOLOGY

Why and when?	Antihistamines are useful in management of allergic conditions in children. Their main indications are **acute allergic reactions**, **allergic rhinitis** (AR) and **chronic spontaneous urticaria** (CSU). The first-generation antihistamines (chlorphenamine, promethazine hydrochloride, ketotifen, hydroxyzine) have lower histamine receptor selectivity and cross the blood–brain barrier leading to **sedative effects**. The second-generation antihistamines (cetirizine, levocetirizine, loratadine, desloratadine, fexofenadine) are preferred due to their duration of action, fewer side effects and safety profile.
Absorption and distribution	There are some differences in absorption and bioavailability of different second-generation antihistamines. Cetirizine has an oral bioavailability of c.70% and levocetirizine an oral bioavailability of c.85% in adults. Cetirizine **poorly crosses the blood–brain barrier** and produces H_1-receptor occupancy levels of about 12% after a single 10 mg dose, **about one-fifth the level achieved with the first-generation antihistamine hydroxyzine**. Oral loratadine and desloratadine are almost completely absorbed (c.100%), but the former is rapidly metabolized in the liver to desloratadine, which is an active metabolite. All achieve peak plasma levels at 1–2 hours and have an onset of action of around 30 minutes. **Fexofenadine has a lower oral bioavailability** (c.35%), a slower peak plasma level (2–3 hours) but lower central nervous system (CNS) penetration.
Biology	Second-generation antihistamines are **selective inverse agonists of peripheral histamine H_1-receptors**. The predicted **potency** of second-generation histamine antagonists is (from strongest to weakest) desloratadine > levocetirizine > cetirizine > fexofenadine > loratadine. However, potency does not correlate well with observed clinical effects and there are significant inter-individual variations in clinical responses to different antihistamines. They competitively block **histamine** receptor sites rather than inhibiting **histamine** release (see chlorphenamine).
Clearance	The elimination half-life of **cetirizine, loratadine and levocetirizine is 8–9 hours** in most adults. Fexofenadine has a half-life of 14–15 hours and desloratadine is much more slowly eliminated, with a half-life of around 27 hours. All have a combination of hepatic and renal clearance mechanisms with the CYP3A4 enzymes being involved in clearance of loratadine and, to a lesser extent, fexofenadine.
	Terminal elimination of antihistamines varies depending on the drug and age of the child. Cetirizine and levocetirizine are eliminated more rapidly in young children where renal clearance is more rapid. This has led to recommendation of twice-daily doses in children up to 6 years of age. Antihistamines are rapidly eliminated from plasma but studies show that a residual effect can occur up to 7 days from H_1-receptor occupancy.

PRACTICAL PRESCRIBING

Dosing	**Cetirizine** 1–2 years: 250 micrograms/kg twice a day 2–6 years: 2.5 mg twice a day 6–12 years: 5 mg twice a day 12–18 years: 10 mg daily **Levocetirizine** 2–6 years: 1.25 mg twice a day 6–18 years: 5 mg once a day **Loratadine** 2–12 years: Child ≤30 kg, 5 mg once a day. Child >30 kg, 10 mg once a day. 12–18 years: 10 mg once a day **Desloratadine** 1–6 years: 1.25 mg once a day 6–12 years: 2.5 mg once a day 12–18 years: 5 mg once a day **Fexofenadine** 6–12 years: 30 mg twice a day 12–18 years: 120 mg once a day (for AR) 12–18 years: 180 mg once a day (for chronic urticarial)
Administration	The most common route of administration of $H_{(1)}$-antihistamines **is oral** but chlorphenamine can be given IV and topical preparations are available for ocular and nasal use. Liquid and tablets forms are available. Tablets are often very small and relatively easy to swallow; they are cheaper and easier to transport than liquid formulations. Most children can be taught to swallow tablets with patience. No parental formulation is available for second-generation antihistamines.
Drug errors and safety	Second-generation antihistamines are all safe and **even at high doses toxicity is limited**. Whilst sedation is common and worse if given in conjunction with other hypnotics, it varies slightly between different antihistamines. In general, fexofenadine produces less sedation with around 15% of adults reporting this compared with c.30% taking cetirizine.
Monitoring	Routine monitoring of blood levels is not required. The efficacy of antihistamines is subjective and is thought to be both patient and disease dependent. Using quality of life measures might give a more accurate determination of antihistamine efficacy in long-term conditions. In clinical practice, many national and international guidelines for chronic urticaria will advocate trials of higher doses, i.e. up to 3 or 4 times the licensed dose.
Cost	Antihistamines are relatively **cheap**. Tablets cost from 2p each (cetirizine 10 mg) to 8p (180 mg fexofenadine). Liquid formulations are a little more expensive, varying from £1 to £10 for 100 mL of the different formulations.

Atenolol

CLINICAL PHARMACOLOGY

Why and when?	Atenolol is a **cardioselective β₁-receptor antagonist**. It is primarily used to treat hypertension and cardiac dysrhythmias. All β-blockers, including atenolol, can induce **bronchospasm** and should be avoided in patients with asthma. One advantage of atenolol, however, is that it has a lesser effect on β₂ bronchial receptors, reducing the impact on the airways.
Absorption and distribution	Atenolol is **fairly well absorbed** from the gastrointestinal tract with a roughly 50% bioavailability. About half an oral dose is excreted unchanged in the faeces. Absorption is reduced by co-administration with food (by around 20%). Following administration on an empty stomach oral atenolol achieves peak concentrations at 2–4 hours. Following absorption atenolol is poorly bound to plasma proteins (3%). It has fewer central nervous system effects than propranolol as it does not easily cross the blood–brain barrier.
Biology	Atenolol binds to **β₁-receptors** on **cardiac smooth muscle and within the kidney.** It blocks the action of noradrenaline. Under most circumstances, the sympathetic nervous system will continuously produce small quantities of noradrenaline, which will act upon adrenoreceptors throughout the body. Atenolol binds to β₁-receptors preventing G protein-stimulated adenyl cyclase conversion of adenosine triphosphate (ATP) into cyclic adenosine monophosphate (cAMP). In the heart this **reduces the force of contraction and speed of conduction**. This reduces blood pressure, cardiac work and oxygen demand. Atenolol also **reduces renin secretion** from the kidney, which is mediated by β₁-receptors. Although atenolol is classified as a cardioselective β₁-receptor antagonist, at higher doses it does have some **β₂-receptor antagonist effects**.
Clearance	Atenolol is eliminated almost entirely **by renal excretion** and has a **plasma half-life of 6–7 hours**. Atenolol is not metabolized extensively and it exerts its pharmacological action on the target receptors without producing metabolites. Its clearance is predictably reduced in individuals with renal failure. In cases of renal impairment doses should be reduced by 50% if eGFR is 10–35 mL/min/1.73 m² and 30–50% of usual dose if eGFR <10 m/min/1.73 m².

PRACTICAL PRESCRIBING

Dosing	For hypertension or cardiac arrhythmias the standard dose for children up to 11 years old is 0.5–2 mg/kg once daily. This may be given as a single dose or in two divided doses. For older children (aged 12–17 years old) the dose is 25 mg–50 mg once daily for treatment of hypertension and 50–100 mg in the treatment of arrhythmias.
Administration	Atenolol is administered orally and is available as tablets. Tablets are available in strengths of 25 mg, 50 mg and 100 mg each. Oral suspension is available in a concentration of 5 mg/mL. Doses should be prescribed in mg and not mL to reduce the error risk.
Side effects and interactions	Atenolol may commonly cause bronchospasm in patients who suffer from asthma. Other side effects include cool peripheries, abdominal discomfort, bradycardia, constipation, dyspnoea, fatigue and headaches. Symptoms that are reversible on discontinuation are those of dry eyes and a rash similar to urticaria. Rarely, it can cause hallucinations and exacerbate psoriasis.

In situations of overdose, presentation includes light-headedness, dizziness and syncope as a result of the resultant bradycardia. Furthermore, this may worsen or precipitate heart failure. |
| Monitoring | It should ideally be avoided in children with asthma. Patients with a history of **obstructive airway disease** require regular **lung function testing.** In clinical practice, the resting heart rate should be taken at each clinical encounter. It should be slow (low end of normal range) once an adequate dose has been achieved but very low heart rates may suggest the need for either a different drug or dose adjustment. |
| Cost | Atenolol is **cheap**. Tablets all cost about 2p each. The cost of oral suspension is a little higher, with prices in the range of £5.60 for 300 mL of the 5 mg/1 mL oral solution. |

Atropine

CLINICAL PHARMACOLOGY

Why and when?	Atropine is a tertiary amine extracted from belladonna alkaloid. It is the prototype of **anticholinergic drugs** but has predominantly **antimuscarinic** effects. It has many uses. It is used in diagnostic eye procedures to evoke mydriasis (dilation of the pupil) and cycloplegia (paralysis of the ciliary muscle of the eye), treatment of bradycardia in cardiovascular scenarios, to reduce salivation and respiratory tract secretions and as an antidote in organophosphorus poisoning. It is an emergency drug and is stocked in resuscitation kits.
Absorption and distribution	Oral atropine is rapidly absorbed after administration with a **bioavailability of about 25%**. It is widely distributed throughout the body and **crosses the blood–brain barrier**. The onset and peak of action depends on the route of administration and the effect sought. The inhibition of salivation after IM administration has an onset within 30 minutes and peak effect at 30–60 minutes. After IV administration the onset is immediate and maximum effect at 0.7–4 minutes.
Biology	Atropine has various effects on different muscarinic receptors of the body, of which the following are of clinical significance.
	Eye: mydriasis, unresponsiveness to light and cycloplegia.
	Cardiovascular: produces divergent effects on the cardiovascular system, depending on the dose. **At low doses**, the predominant effect is a **slight decrease in heart rate** because of blockade of M1 receptors on the inhibitory prejunctional neurons, thus permitting increased acetylcholine release. **Higher doses of atropine cause a progressive increase in heart rate** by blocking M2 receptors on the sinoatrial node.
	Secretions: atropine blocks muscarinic receptors in the salivary glands, producing **dryness of the mouth**. The salivary glands are exquisitely sensitive to atropine and 1% eye drops given orally (under the tongue) can dramatically reduce salivation, although it is unlicensed for this indication. Sweat and lacrimal glands are similarly affected. Inhibition of secretions of sweat glands can cause elevated body temperature, which can be dangerous in children and the elderly.
Clearance	Atropine is distributed throughout the tissues. Compartmental clearance can be delayed. Applied to eyes, it freely penetrates cornea and the effect **may persist for days**. Some of the drug is destroyed by enzymatic hydrolysis, particularly in the liver, but the majority is eliminated renally. About 50% is excreted unchanged in the urine. It has a plasma half-life of about **2 hours** in adults but is slightly prolonged in younger children.

PRACTICAL PRESCRIBING

Dosing	Available as 600 microgram (mcg) tablets, 1% eye drops (1 drop provides c.0.5 mg) and solution for injection in various strengths either as pre-filled syringes or as ampoules.
	Cycloplegia: apply 1 eye drop to each eye twice daily for 3 days before procedure.
	Anterior uveitis: apply 1 drop to affected eye(s) four times a day.
	Bradycardia due to overdosage of β-blockers: **40 mcg/kg** by **IV injection** (max. 3 mg)
	Organophosphorus poisoning (in combination with pralidoxime): **20 mcg/kg by IV injection** (max. 2 mg) **every 5–10 minutes** until the skin becomes flushed and dry, the pupils dilate, and the bradycardia is abolished.
	Premedication before anaesthesia: to be given IV immediately before induction of anaesthesia.
	Neonate: 10 mcg/kg. Children 1 month–11 yrs: **20 mcg/kg** (min. 100 mcg, max. 600 mcg). Children >12 yrs: 300–600 mcg.
Administration	For IV route, to be administered undiluted by **rapid IV injection** as slow injection may result in paradoxical bradycardia. In children, injection solution may be given orally. If eye drops are used to reduce drooling then 1 or 2 drops are usually used every 4–6 hours. The latter is an unlicensed indication.
Drug errors and safety	Eye drops should not be used in children below 3 months, owing to possible association between **cycloplegia and the amblyopia**. Also the use of eye drops may precipitate **acute angle closure glaucoma**. Oral atropine will have many **predictable dose-dependent side effects** including gastrointestinal dysfunction, abdominal distension, anhidrosis, anxiety, blurred vision, dysphagia, taste loss and thirst.
Monitoring	In some circumstances and after IV use, heart rate, blood pressure, pulse and mental status monitoring is required. During administration for organophosphorus poisoning, monitor for signs and symptoms of atropine toxicity (fever, muscle fasciculation, delirium); if it occurs, discontinue it. **After oral or topical administration monitoring is not usually indicated** but doses may need to be adjusted according to clinical response.
Cost	Atropine is **fairly expensive**. 600 mcg tablets cost almost £2 each. 10 mL of 1% eye drops costs c.£130 and 3 mg of IV atropine costs £7–8. IV forms may be given orally. Minims® atropine sulfate 1% eye drops are a little less expensive and cost c.75p for 0.5 mL units.

Azithromycin

CLINICAL PHARMACOLOGY

Why and when?

Azithromycin is a widely used antibiotic in the paediatric population. It is used to treat conditions such as chest infection, throat, skin, ear infection and some sexually transmitted diseases. In most of the cases, it is used as a second-line antibiotic or acts as an adjunct to other antibiotics. In many instances it works as a substitute for patients with penicillin allergy. It is commonly used as a prophylactic antibiotic in children with chronic respiratory diseases and has a good evidence base for use as a **prophylactic treatment in children over 6 years with cystic fibrosis**. Some recent studies have shown effectiveness as a treatment for acute asthma exacerbations in children. However, it is not widely used (or recommended) for this indication due to concerns about emergence of antibiotic resistance. Azithromycin is dispensed as liquid, tablet, capsule, eye drop forms.

Absorption and distribution

Oral azithromycin is rapidly absorbed from the gastrointestinal tract. Food hinders its absorption and reduces bioavailability of capsules but probably not other formulations. Magnesium and aluminium hydroxide antacids also decrease serum peak concentrations. It poorly concentrates in cerebrospinal fluid but has otherwise wide tissue distribution among tissues and cells. It generally achieves very high tissue concentrations and fibroblasts work as a natural reservoir *in vivo*. Serum concentrations are generally much lower than tissue concentrations. Human polymorphonuclear **leucocytes achieve up to 300-fold the extracellular concentration** of azithromycin, where it is stored within lysosomes. Its oral bioavailability is 34–52%. 50% is bound to protein at very low plasma concentration and even lower in higher concentrations. Peak onset of action is around 2–3 hours following an oral dose.

Biology

Azithromycin is a semisynthetic derivative of erythromycin. It contains 15-membered lactone rings to which attach deoxy sugars in comparison to the 14-membered ringed parent molecule erythromycin. Azithromycin has one extra methyl-substituted nitrogen atom into the lactone ring. These alterations improved acid **stability**, **tissue penetration** and broad-spectrum **activity** when compared with erythromycin.

Like other members of the macrolide group of antibiotics, it acts as a **bacteriostatic** agent. Azithromycin inhibits mRNA transcription and thereby prevents protein synthesis by binding to 50S ribosomal subunits of sensitive bacteria.

Azithromycin is effective against most *Staphylococcus* and *Streptococcus* species. It is also very effective for *Mycoplasma*, *Chlamydia*, *Moraxella*, *Legionella*, *Bordetella*, *Borrelia* and *Helicobacter pylori*. It has enhanced action against mycobacterium avium-complex and few protozoa (*Toxoplasma*, cryptosporidium and *Plasmodium* species). Although effective, it is not the drug of choice for *Haemophilus*. It is not useful for enteric Gram-negative bacilli. It must be used very judiciously in order to curb rising **problems of drug resistance.**

PRACTICAL PRESCRIBING

Clearance	Biliary excretion is the major route of elimination, however some metabolism happens in liver as well, giving rise to inactive metabolites. Only 12–14% is excreted unchanged in urine. It has a prolonged elimination half-life (40–68 hours) due to extensive tissue distribution and binding.
Dosing	Azithromycin dose in paediatric population is age, weight and disease dependent. In most common circumstances a dose of 10 mg/kg is appropriate with a maximum daily dose of 500 mg. Due to its unique characteristics it is given **once a day for 3 days at the same time to treat acute infections and 3 times a week when used as prophylaxis**. The reduced frequency of dosing and relatively low incidence of side effects result in better compliance than other macrolides.
Administration	Azithromycin capsules should be given 1 hour before or 2 hours after meals when administered orally. Patients need to swallow whole tablets or capsules with a glass of water. Liquid for children is usually made up by pharmacists and should come with a syringe. Missed doses should be taken as soon as possible. Patients report **significant differences in the palatability of different brands**.
Drug errors and safety	Azithromycin is a relatively safe drug. Mild side effects can be seen in 1 in 100 people. Most common complaints are nausea, vomiting, diarrhoea, loss of appetite, rash, tiredness and dizziness. Serious side effects are rare (<1 in 1000). In children with diabetes it should be used cautiously as oral suspensions often contain sugar. In case of renal or hepatic impairment, dose should be reduced. All macrolides should be used with caution in patients with a predisposition to QT interval prolongation. It is generally not recommended in pregnancy, although it can be taken if benefits outweigh the risk and must be discussed with a doctor. It does not interact with alcohol or oral contraceptives.
Monitoring	Efficacy of azithromycin should be measured with signs of improvement of symptoms. Routine blood monitoring is not required.
Cost	Azithromycin is **costlier than many other antibiotics**. But its use is rising sharply due to unique effectiveness and better compliance with a once-daily regimen. Oral tablets are much cheaper than syrup. 1 g tablets roughly cost around £1.12, whereas oral suspension costs £11.04 for 1.2 g. Once the oral solution has been reconstituted it has a relatively short 'shelf-life' of just 5 days, which can be very frustrating and difficult for families taking longer-term treatment. Some individuals will be provided with powder for reconstitution at home.

Baclofen

CLINICAL PHARMACOLOGY

Why and when?	Baclofen is a γ-aminobutyric acid (GABA) agonist used as a **skeletal muscle relaxant.** It is used for the relief of painful and uncomfortable muscle **spasms of cerebral origin**, such as cerebral palsy. It is also used in **disorders of spinal cord** and **multiple sclerosis**. Baclofen improves mobility, increasing levels of independence, and facilitates physiotherapy. Children receiving this drug should have reversible spasticity.
Absorption and distribution	Baclofen is **rapidly absorbed** from the gastrointestinal tract with a **bioavailability of 70–80%**. Absorption may be dose dependent, as it reduces with increasing doses. Baclofen **does not readily cross the blood–brain barrier**, with cerebrospinal fluid (CSF) concentrations of about 12% of the plasma concentration following oral administration. 30% is bound to plasma proteins.
Biology	Baclofen is an effective and widely used antispastic agent with a **spinal site of action**. In addition, baclofen has other central sites of action, shown by its adverse event profile and general central nervous system (CNS) depressant properties. Neuroimaging studies in humans indicate that baclofen produces region-specific alterations in brain activity. It stimulates gastric acid secretion.
	The exact mechanism of action of baclofen is not fully understood. Baclofen **depresses monosynaptic and polysynaptic reflex transmission** by various actions, and possibly including the stimulation of $GABA_B$-receptors. This stimulation results in the **inhibition of excitatory neurotransmitter** (glutamate and aspartate) release, which may normally contribute to pain and spasticity. It relieves spasms and associated pain and clonus, in addition to muscular rigidity.
Clearance	Following oral administration, peak concentrations occur in about 1–3 hours. The **half-life of baclofen is about 5 hours**. It is rapidly excreted from the body, with **70–80% excreted by the kidneys** as unchanged drug. The remainder of the drug is excreted either unchanged in faeces or as inactive metabolites in faeces and urine. Excretion is complete within 3 days. There is a marked variation in elimination rates between patients.

Intrathecal baclofen

Baclofen, when introduced directly into the intrathecal space, allows for effective CSF concentrations to be achieved, with resulting plasma concentrations 100 times less than concentrations occurring with oral administration. This can be done using a baclofen pump with an intrathecal catheter inserted. Great care needs to be taken in assessing children receiving intrathecal baclofen as abrupt cessation can be dangerous. The symptoms of pump failure are initially non-specific but include increased distress and spasm.

PRACTICAL PRESCRIBING

Dosing	For **oral** administration, drug is introduced at a dose of **300 micrograms (mcg)/kg/day** in 4 divided doses in children ≥1 month of age. The dose is gradually increased as weekly increments until a satisfactory clinical response is achieved. The **maintenance dose is 0.75–2 mg/kg/day** in divided doses with a maximum of 40 mg/day (60 mg/day in children ≥8 years). Treatment should be reviewed if there is no benefit within 6 weeks after achieving maximum dose. The **intrathecal** route can be used in **children ≥4 years** of age where oral treatment has been ineffective, was not tolerated or is not possible. A test dose of **25–50 mcg** is given over 1 minute via a catheter or lumbar puncture. The dose is initially increased by **increments of 25 mcg** (max 100 mcg) at **minimum 24-hour intervals** to determine the maintenance dose. **Maintenance dose is usually 25–200 mcg/day** and is adjusted according to response. The maintenance dose is titrated, usually using an infusion pump, to retain some spasticity to avoid sensation of paralysis.
Side effects and considerations	Side effects include dry mouth, nausea, vomiting, diarrhoea, constipation, skin reactions, paraesthesia, headache, dizziness, drowsiness, confusion, hallucination, depression, euphoria, hyperhidrosis, hypotension, urinary disorders, vision disorders, bradycardia, hypothermia, fatigue, muscle weakness, myalgia, respiratory depression and sleep disorders. **Intrathecal use** can cause anxiety, decreased appetite, pain, fever, chills, hypersalivation, insomnia, neuromuscular dysfunction, oedema, respiratory disorders, seizure and sexual dysfunction. Care should be taken to check medicine supply in the pump and malfunction if side effects occur. **Peptic ulceration** is a contraindication to the oral use of medicine. Intrathecal route is contraindicated in local or systemic **infection**, while it should be used with caution in **coagulation disorders**, **post-spinal surgery** and malnutrition. Doses should be **adjusted in renal failure**. It should be used with caution in liver failure, diabetes, epilepsy, psychiatric illness, hypertonic bladder sphincter and respiratory impairment. It should be **avoided in pregnancy**. It is secreted in breast milk although the amount is very small and unlikely to be harmful. Treatment **should not be discontinued abruptly** (withdrawal symptoms, including hallucinations and seizures). It should be **tapered over a period of at least 1–2 weeks**. **Patient information for parents** is available at https://www.medicinesforchildren.org.uk/baclofen-muscle-spasm.
Cost	Oral treatment is cost effective with the oral solution available as 5 mg/5 mL formulation (300 mL) being charged at £1.40 for 100 mL and tablets available as 10 mg (pack of 84) with each costing 1.4 p. Solution for infusion is available in different strengths (10 mg/5 mL, 10 mg/20 mL, 40 mg/20 mL), and 10 mg of infusion medicine costs approximately £50–60. There are also additional costs for the device and insertion, along with monitoring by specialist nurses regularly who refill the device.

Beclometasone dipropionate

CLINICAL PHARMACOLOGY

Why and when?

Beclometasone is a synthetic corticosteroid. It is used in the treatment and **prophylaxis of asthma** as either an inhaled powder or, more commonly in children, as a pressurized metered-dose inhaler (pMDI) with valved-holding chamber (spacer). It is used with the aim of preventing asthma exacerbations and not in the management of acute asthma. Beclometasone is also used in the treatment and prophylaxis of **allergic rhinitis** (including hay fever) and severe **inflammatory skin disorders** unresponsive to less potent corticosteroids.

Absorption

When administered via an inhaler, some beclometasone dipropionate (BDP) is deposited directly into the lungs and absorbed into the systemic circulation. BDP is a prodrug. Prior to absorption there is extensive hydrolysis of BDP via tissue esterases, which are present in most of the body, to its active metabolite beclometasone-17-monopropionate (B-17-MP).

Whilst a variably large proportion of inhaled BDP is swallowed (40–60%), there is relatively lower bioavailability from oral absorption of the swallowed dose (c.25% for B-17-MP), leading to less systemic absorption and some reduction in systemic side effects. The systemic absorption of B-17-MP from the lungs is higher (36–41%) and due to its location of absorption will not undergo first-pass metabolism. This results in an absolute bioavailability of c.60% for B-17-MP, following inhalation. The effective dose is therefore highly dependent upon **inhalation technique**, the age and size of **the child**, the use (or not) of a **valved-holding chamber** (spacer) and **the particle size** delivered. Whilst inhaled doses result in less adrenal suppression and fewer side effects than oral steroids, daily doses in excess of 800 micrograms (mcg) (400 mcg of ultrafine particle Qvar®) are likely to lead to adrenal suppression.

Biology

BDP acts as an anti-inflammatory mainly via its metabolite, B-17-MP. B-17-MP has a 25-times greater affinity for the glucocorticoid receptor than BDP. Unbound B-17-MP binds to cell surface receptor and is internalized. Beclometasone then binds to specific glucocorticoid receptors. These steroid-receptor complexes act in the nucleus leading to altered gene expression and inhibition of pro-inflammatory cytokine production. The **exact mechanism of action is not fully understood** but includes inhibition of inflammatory cells and inflammatory mediators. These are all thought to play a role in the anti-inflammatory and immunomodulatory effects. Clinically this translates to reduction in oedema, inflammation and scar tissue.

Clearance

BDP is cleared very rapidly following metabolism by esterases. Beclometasone and its metabolites have high plasma clearance (150 L/hour and 120 L/hour) and a terminal elimination half-life of 0.5 to 2.8 hours for BDP and B-17-MP, respectively. It is excreted mainly in the faeces regardless of administration route (inhalation, oral, injection or topical). Less than 10% of beclometasone or its metabolites are excreted in the urine.

PRACTICAL PRESCRIBING

Dosing	In the management of asthma, inhaled beclometasone doses **start at 100 mcg twice daily** and increase up to maximum of 800 mcg twice a day. Combination inhalers are available which contain BDP and long-acting β_2-agonists, at varying doses, although **most are currently unlicensed for children under 12**. For the prophylaxis and treatment of allergic rhinitis in children over the age of 6 years the usual topical dose is **100 mcg twice daily** via nasal spray; this should be reduced when symptoms are controlled. Care must be taken when using both inhalers and nasal sprays as the potential for adrenal suppression is increased. For eczema and psoriasis a thin layer of beclometasone ointment 0.025% should be used 1–2 times daily. This should be applied using the 'fingertip unit' method (see hydrocortisone).
Administration	Inhalation via CFC-free pMDI, dry powder inhaler (DPI), nasal spray or topically, using cream. Beclometasone-only inhalers include Clenil modulite® and Qvar®. **These are not interchangeable** and should be prescribed using their brand name. Qvar has extra-fine particles that are delivered more efficiently to the lung and therefore it is considered to be twice as potent. **pMDIs should be used in conjunction with spacer devices in children**.
Drug errors and safety	Acute toxicity is low, but in common with all corticosteroids, **suppression of hypothalamic-pituitary-adrenal function is well recognized** and this should be screened for clinically, particularly in children receiving higher doses (>400 mcg of BDP per day). Children on higher doses should carry a steroid card warning against abrupt withdrawal and giving advice about illness or chickenpox exposure. Other corticosteroid-associated adverse effects, including cataract, glaucoma and decrease in bone density, are very rarely seen with inhalation; by contrast hoarseness, throat irritation and oral candidiasis are common and very common. Following environmental concerns chlorofluorocarbons (CFCs) were removed from many products, including pMDIs. CFCs were replaced with hydrofluoroalkane (HFA)-powered MDIs and this resulted in an unexpected improvement of small particle delivery to the lower respiratory tract with less deposition in the oropharynx and less systematic absorption.
Monitoring	No official drug level monitoring is done for patients taking beclometasone in any of its forms, but **growth and height velocity** in particular **should be carefully monitored** in any child on long-term inhaled corticosteroids (see fluticasone for more details).
Cost	Most BDP preparations **are cheap** when compared with other inhaled or nasal steroids. A 200-dose bottle of nasal spray costs c.£3 and a 200-dose 50 mcg/actuation pMDI costs £3–4 (double for Qvar). Skin creams, by comparison with other topical steroids, are relatively expensive (c.£70 for 30 g).

Calcium

CLINICAL PHARMACOLOGY

Why and when?	Calcium is necessary for normal functioning of nerves, cells, muscle and bone. Almost 99% of total body calcium is found in the skeleton, with only small amounts found in the plasma and extravascular fluid. Calcium as an oral supplement is used often in conjunction with vitamin D to prevent calcium deficiency in children who either do not absorb enough or who do not get enough calcium from their diets. Parenteral calcium salts (calcium gluconate) are used in treating **acute hypocalcaemia** and calcium is used to reduce the risk of cardiac arrhythmias in **hyperkalaemia**. Calcium salt is also used to treat **hyperphosphatemia** in patients with chronic kidney disease by combining with dietary phosphate to form insoluble calcium phosphate, which is excreted in faeces.
Absorption and reabsorption	Calcium is absorbed by facilitated diffusion from the entire small intestine as well as from the duodenum by a carrier-mediated active transport system **under the influence of vitamin D**. Only one-third of orally ingested calcium is absorbed. However, fractional absorption of calcium is greater in the presence of calcium deficiency and low dietary calcium. Phytates, phosphates, oxalates and tetracyclines bind calcium in an insoluble form and reduce absorption. **Glucocorticoids and phenytoin** also **reduce calcium absorption**.
	Ionized calcium is **totally filtered at the glomerulus** and most of it is reabsorbed in the tubules. Vitamin D and parathyroid hormone increase and calcitonin decreases tubular reabsorption of calcium.
Biology	Calcium is an **integral component of the skeleton** and also moderates nerve and muscle performance and allows normal cardiac function. Calcium carbonate as a dietary supplement is used to prevent or treat negative calcium balance; in osteoporosis, it helps to prevent or decrease the rate of bone loss.
	Calcium salts act as antacids neutralizing gastric acidity resulting in increased gastric and duodenal bulb pH. They will inhibit the proteolytic activity of pepsin if the pH is increased >4 and increase lower oesophageal sphincter tone.
Clearance	In adults about **300 mg of endogenous calcium is excreted daily:** half in urine and half in faeces. To maintain calcium balance, the same amount has to be absorbed in the small intestine from the diet. **Thiazide diuretics impede calcium excretion** by facilitating tubular reabsorption. 80% of insoluble calcium salts are excreted through faeces and 20% through urine.

PRACTICAL PRESCRIBING

Dosing	Oral calcium salts are used to treat calcium deficiency.
	The dose **is 0.25 mmol/kg four times** a day for children <5 years, **0.2 mmol/kg four times** a day for children 5–11 years and **10 mmol four times a day** for 12–17-year-olds.
	Intravenous calcium gluconate is used for acute hypocalcaemia, urgent correction and hyperkalaemia.
	The dose is **0.11 mmol/kg/dose**, which is to be given over 5–10 minutes (maximum 4.5 mmol). 0.11 mmol/kg is equivalent to **0.5 mL/kg of calcium gluconate 10%**. Calcium gluconate is also used for maintenance therapy as a continuous intravenous infusion.
Administration	Calcium is available in various forms as salts combined with other elements, which differ in the amount of calcium they contain. It is available as calcium carbonate, calcium lactate, calcium acetate, calcium citrate, calcium gluconate, calcium phosphate, calcium chloride and calcium citrate.
	The most commonly available calcium salt forms are calcium carbonate and calcium citrate. Oral calcium is widely available in a range of formulations and concentrations. These include tablets, capsules and oral suspensions that are available over the counter. It is available in IV forms as 10% solutions for injection in 10 mL ampoules.
Drug errors and safety	The potential side effects of oral calcium are constipation, diarrhoea, hypercalcaemia and nausea. **Calcium carbonate at high doses** can cause hypercalciuria leading to **kidney stones**. Very rarely it causes flatulence, gastrointestinal discomfort, milk-alkali syndrome and skin reactions. With IV use calcium gluconate can cause arrhythmias, shock, hyperhidrosis, hypotension, vasodilatation and vomiting.
Monitoring	All calcium salts should be used with caution in view of hypercalciuria and renal calculi. Hence **regular serum calcium monitoring is important to avoid calcium toxicity** after starting calcium supplements or intravenous calcium infusion. It is important to monitor plasma and urinary calcium during long-term maintenance therapy.
Cost	Calcium is **fairly cheap**. 10 mL of calcium gluconate solution for injection 10% costs £0.75. Calcium carbonate is available as effervescent and chewable tablets. The cost of a 500 mg effervescent tablet is 15p and for a 500 mg chewable tablet it is 6p.

Captopril

CLINICAL PHARMACOLOGY

Why and when?	Captopril is an angiotensin-converting enzyme (ACE) inhibitor. It slows the conversion of angiotensin I to its biologically active form angiotensin II, which has several important biological actions. One of its main clinical applications is to treat **hypertension and congestive heart failure**. It also acts to decrease glomerular filtration rate and is used to manage proteinuria secondary to nephritis, including diabetic nephropathy.
Absorption and distribution	Captopril is well absorbed from the upper gastrointestinal tract with an estimated bioavailability of 70% but co-administration with food decreases its absorption. Absorption is rapid with onset of action at 15 minutes after administration. Protein binding is 25–30%.
Biology	Captopril competitively inhibits ACE, preventing the conversion of angiotensin I to angiotensin II, a potent vasoconstrictor. ACE inhibitors therefore **decrease vascular resistance** (afterload) and venous tone (preload). This reduction of systemic vascular resistance will decrease blood pressure and **increase cardiac output** *if* there is excessive afterload and **adequate preload**. The main biological functions of angiotensin II are summarized below:

Blood vessels	Vasoconstriction
Kidney	↑ Na+ reabsorption
Sympathetic nervous system	↑ noradrenaline release
Adrenal cortex	↑ aldosterone secretion
Hypothalamus	↑ thirst, ↑ anti-diuretic hormone

	Its vasodilator action involves the efferent arteriole of the glomerulus, resulting in decreased glomerular filtration rate. ACE is very similar to endogenous enzymes that break down bradykinin, which is also vasoactive and this may explain some of its side effects.
Clearance	In contrast to most of the drugs of its class, captopril is not a prodrug. The **half-life is 3.3 hours** in infants and **1.5 hours in children**. It is largely (>95%) excreted in the urine, 40–50% as unchanged drug.
Dosing	The dose is dependent on age, weight and renal function. Captopril may cause **profound hypotension** even in small doses and a tolerability test is mandatory upon initiation. Administration of test dose is followed by 1–2 hours of blood pressure monitoring. The **test dose** is 10–50 micrograms (mcg)/kg for neonates and 100 mcg/kg for infants and children (maximum test dose is 6.25 mg).

PRACTICAL PRESCRIBING

Dosing (continued)	The usual starting dose is 10–50 mcg/kg for neonates, 100–300 mcg/kg for infants and children under 12 and 12.5–25 mg for children older than 12 years. The dose is given **2–3 times/day** and increased as necessary. The total daily dose for captopril can reach up to 300 mcg/kg for preterm, 2 mg/kg for term neonates, 4 mg/kg for infants and 6 mg/kg for children (maximum daily dose is 150 mg). Captopril should be used with extreme caution in those with impaired renal function and careful titration is essential, often with monitoring in the hospital setting.
Administration	Captopril is administered orally and is available as tablets and oral solution. Tablets are available in strengths of 12.5 mg, 25 mg and 50 mg each. Oral solution exists in strengths of 5 mg/5 mL and 25 mg/5 mL. Tablets can be dispersed in water. The first dose of captopril should be ideally given at bedtime. There is a high risk of medication errors due to there being two strengths of oral liquid available; care must be taken when prescribing.
Side effects and interactions	Captopril may cause symptomatic **hypotension** and syncope. Patients on high doses of diuretics, a low-sodium diet, dialysis, are dehydrated, have heart failure or those with severe or symptomatic aortic stenosis are at higher risk. Captopril may also induce **renal failure** and hyperkalaemia due to reduction in glomerular filtration rate and aldosterone activity. The risk is increased in those with impaired renal function. **Its use is contraindicated in patients with bilateral renovascular disease**. Captopril may cause hypoglycaemia and caution is advised when it is administered to diabetic patients. Captopril can, rarely, cause haemolytic anaemia and neutropenia, and, also rarely, hepatotoxicity.
	Persistent **dry cough** is a particular fairly common problem with all ACE inhibitors; more rarely, ACE inhibitors may cause serious hypersensitivity reactions including **angioedema** and **Stevens–Johnson** syndrome or **anaphylactoid** reactions. Angioedema may be delayed and occur at any point after initiation of treatment. Afro-Caribbean patients are at higher risk. Neonates are more sensitive to side effects. ACE inhibitors are teratogenic and should be avoided in pregnancy. Their use should be avoided by breastfeeding mothers during the first few weeks after delivery.
	The risk for hypotension, hyperkalaemia and renal failure is increased when captopril is combined with other drugs with similar pharmacological effects, such as antihypertensives and diuretics.
Monitoring	**Renal function and electrolytes should be checked** before starting ACE inhibitors (or increasing the dose) and monitored during treatment.
Cost	Oral solutions are **relatively expensive** and vary between £98 (5 mg/mL) and £109 (25 mg/mL) for 100 mL. Tablets are cheaper and vary between £0.79 and £1.92 for packs of 56 tablets.

Carbamazepine

CLINICAL PHARMACOLOGY

Why and when?	Carbamazepine, one of the most widely used **antiepileptic drugs**, is chemically related to the tricyclic antidepressant drugs and was found in a routine screening test to inhibit electrically evoked seizures in mice. Pharmacologically and clinically, its actions resemble those of **phenytoin** and **lamotrigine**, although it appears to be particularly effective in treating certain **partial seizures** with or without secondary generalization. It is also first-line treatment for **trigeminal neuralgia** and to treat other conditions, such as **neuropathic pain** and manic-depressive illness. It is not recommended for primary generalized seizures (especially myoclonic epilepsy, which can be worsened by it).
Absorption	Carbamazepine is relatively slowly but well absorbed (75–80%) after oral administration. Its absorption is not reduced by food. It is mostly (c.75%) protein bound and distributes widely throughout the tissues. It crosses the blood–brain barrier and the placenta and cerebrospinal fluid (CSF) concentrations are very similar to unbound serum levels (c.25% of total serum value). Oral **suspension reaches peak** concentration much **more rapidly** than tablet forms (c.1.5 hours compared to 4–5 hours). Therefore, peak levels may be higher with suspension dosing and the dose may need to be lowered.
Biology	Carbamazepine exerts its effects mainly by action on **voltage-gated sodium channels**. These are expressed throughout the neuron and are responsible for depolarization and conduction of action potentials. There is a use-dependent **blockade** of voltage-gated Na channels, which inhibits repetitive neuronal firing. There is also an attenuation of the action of glutamate at N-methyl-D-aspartate **(NMDA) receptors**, which leads to **reduced glutamate release**. Carbamazepine is a powerful **inducer of hepatic microsomal enzymes** and thus accelerates the metabolism of many other drugs, such as phenytoin, oral contraceptives, warfarin and corticosteroids, as well as of itself.
Clearance	Carbamazepine is eliminated following metabolism in the **liver**. Whilst carbamazepine metabolites are renally excreted (c.75%) only a very small amount is excreted unchanged in the urine (c.1%). **Hepatic enzyme activity** varies between individuals and over time and is influenced by carbamazepine itself and other medicines. In general, it is inadvisable to combine it with other antiepileptic drugs, and interactions with other drugs (e.g. warfarin) metabolized by cytochrome P450 (CYP) enzymes are common and clinically important.

The half-life of carbamazepine falls from approximately 36 hours to 12–18 hours over the first few weeks of therapy due to **autoinduction** of hepatic enzymes. For this reason, **the dose is gradually increased** over many weeks with the intention that plasma levels will remain within therapeutic range over time. Once absorbed, carbamazepine is metabolized by the liver to an epoxide; both compounds possess antiepileptic activity, but the epoxide may cause more adverse effects. |

PRACTICAL PRESCRIBING

Dosing	When starting treatment, the opposite of a 'loading dose' strategy is employed: **small initial doses are gradually increased**. As enzyme induction occurs, increasing doses are needed to maintain therapeutic plasma concentrations. For seizure disorder, prophylaxis of bipolar disorder and trigeminal neuralgia the doses are age and weight dependent. In children under 12 then a typical starting dose is 5 mg/kg once daily (at night) or 2.5 mg/kg twice daily. This is then increased in steps of 2.5–5 mg/kg every 3–7 days as required. The **usual maintenance dose is 5 mg/kg 2–3 times a day**, increased if necessary up to 20 mg/kg daily. For older children and adults, initial doses are 100–200 mg, 1–2 times a day. This is increased to 200–400 mg, 2–3 times a day, increased slowly if necessary up to 1.8 g daily. If oral administration is not possible, a **rectal formulation** is available for short-term use (max. 7 days). It is usually necessary to use approximately 25% more than the oral dose.
Side effects and considerations for use	**Drug interaction and enzyme induction are common** and care must be taken when using other drugs. Common side effects are best remembered as being **peripheral** (skin reactions, dry mouth, hyponatraemia and oedema), **central** (ataxia, blurred vision, dizziness, drowsiness, fatigue, headache, nausea and vomiting) and **blood disorders** (anaemia, thrombocytopenia, eosinophilia). Care should be taken when switching between different oral formulations in the treatment of epilepsy. The MHRA recommends for carbamazepine that the patient should be maintained on a **specific manufacturer's brand** and the **prescription should specify this**.
	Other drugs relying on hepatic metabolism may also have their **effective plasma level decreased** due to induction secondary to carbamazepine, e.g. glucocorticosteroids, contraceptive pill, theophylline, warfarin, as well as other anticonvulsants, e.g. phenytoin. The metabolism of carbamazepine itself may be inhibited by valproate and, to a lesser extent, by lamotrigine and levetiracetam (thereby raising carbamazepine plasma levels). Oxcarbazepine is a prodrug that is metabolized to a compound closely resembling carbamazepine with similar actions but there is a lesser tendency to induce drug-metabolizing enzymes.
Monitoring	There is a recommendation that blood counts and hepatic/renal function should be monitored but evidence of practical value is uncertain.
Cost	Oral forms of carbamazepine, including modified-release preparations are **relatively cheap**. Oral carbamazepine suspension is available in the strength 100 mg/5 mL. It costs approximately £7 for 300 mL. Tablets and modified-release tablets are available as 100 mg, 200 mg and 400 mg and cost 3–20p each depending upon strength and precise formulation. The **suppository is expensive** costing £24–28 for a single 125 mg/250 mg dose.

Carobel

CLINICAL PHARMACOLOGY

Why and when?	Carobel is a feed thickener that has a proven efficacy in the treatment of **gastroesophageal reflux disease** (GORD) in infants. There are several thickeners available including carob bean gum, rice cereal, corn starch or alginates. Thickeners do reduce the frequency of regurgitation in infants with proven GORD but the effects on other symptoms such as faltering growth, irritability and respiratory symptoms are unproven.
	The active ingredient in Carobel is **locust bean gum**. This is a galactomannan vegetable gum extracted from the seeds of the carob tree. It consists chiefly of high-molecular-weight hydrocolloidal polysaccharides, composed of galactose and mannose units combined through glycosidic linkages. It is a common food additive (**E410**) and usually well tolerated.
Absorption	Carobel is almost **completely absorbed in the small intestine**. Most of the calories are delivered as carbohydrates. All carbohydrates absorbed in the small intestine must be hydrolyzed to monosaccharides prior to absorption. Unabsorbed locust bean gum has the potential to thicken the stool and may result in constipation.
Biology	Carobel contains a significant number of calories, which can be particularly helpful if a child has previously had faltering growth. A single scoop **contains 5.4 kCal** and usually a scoop is added to approximately 58 mL (2 fluid ounces) of formula. This can make a significant difference to weight gain as if used with every feed and standard infant formula it **increases the calorific content by about 15%**. Carobel contains small amounts of other minerals and nutrients. It has a significant amount of calcium and will add about 20% to the calcium intake of a formula-fed baby of less than 3 months of age.
Clearance	Carobel and its components are subject to **extensive post-absorption metabolism**. It is mostly carbohydrate but contains a small amount of fat and no protein. In addition to calcium, it contains small amounts of sodium, chloride and potassium. Each scoop contains 1.5 mg of potassium (about 0.025 mmol). This is not usually of any clinical significance.

PRACTICAL PRESCRIBING

Dosing	Carobel can be added to infant formula or mixed to form a paste, which is given prior to feeds. When added to formula it is most usual to recommend a single scoop (1.7 g) to each feed. The maximum recommended concentration is 3%, which is one scoop to 2 fluid ounces (58.8 mL) of infant formula. Lower concentrations (as low as one scoop for 150 mL of infant formula) can still be effective. After mixing with the infant formula it is necessary to let the mixture stand for 3–4 minutes. The bottle must then be shaken well before giving it to the baby. Once mixed it will continue to thicken for 10–15 minutes. When used in breastfed infants, a gel can be prepared by adding three level scoops of Carobel to 60 mL of warm, previously boiled water. After mixing with vigorous stirring it should be allowed to thicken for 3–4 minutes before stirring again and spoon-feeding to the baby.
Administration	Locust bean gum is palatable. Indeed, it is often used as a food additive because it is sweet. Most babies will take it with little encouragement. When used with infant formula, adding a scoop to 60 mL of infant formula will result in a 3% solution. The increased viscosity can lead to blockage of the teat.
Drug errors and safety	Although Carobel is considered safe in term infants, there are concerns that its use in preterm infants may **increase the risk of necrotizing enterocolitis**.
Monitoring	Routine monitoring is not required. Parents should be warned that all feed thickeners may alter the appearance and consistency of the stool and may result in constipation.
Cost	Carobel is fairly cheap. 135 g (about 80 doses) costs around £3. This will be enough to last most babies under 3 months for about a week. It can also be bought over the counter by parents.

Cefotaxime

CLINICAL PHARMACOLOGY

Why and when?	Cefotaxime is a third-generation cephalosporin **antibiotic**. It has a broad spectrum of activity (Gram-negative and Gram-positive) but is **particularly potent** against β-lactamase-producing **Gram-negative organisms**. It is **bactericidal.** It has limited activity against *Pseudomonas aeruginosa*. It crosses the blood–brain barrier when the meninges are inflamed and is therefore a first-line treatment for Gram-negative meningitis. It has a similar efficacy and safety profile to ceftriaxone but its shorter duration of action means it has to be given more frequently. It is often **used empirically** as a broad-spectrum antibiotic in a child **with suspected septicaemia or meningitis**.
Absorption and distribution	Cefotaxime is **not absorbed from the gastrointestinal tract** and therefore must be given intravenously or by intramuscular (IM) injection. Both the intravenous (IV) and IM routes lead to good bioavailability (>90%) and this is not significantly reduced by co-administration with lignocaine when given IM. Following IV administration it is distributed **widely to most body tissues and fluids**. 13–38% is protein bound.
Biology	Cefotaxime is a **β-lactam antibiotic**. It belongs to the class of organic compounds known as cephalosporin 3'-esters. These are cephalosporins that are esterified at the 3'-position. Its structure means it is **resistant to the effects of β-lactamase**. Cefotaxime exerts its **bactericidal action** by inhibiting bacterial cell wall synthesis. It binds to **penicillin-binding proteins** in the cell wall and inhibits peptidoglycan cross linkage. The bacterium is then killed by osmotic lysis. As with other β-lactam antibiotics, cefotaxime exhibits time-dependent killing. This means the key pharmacodynamic parameter in determining its antimicrobial effect is the time that serum concentration remains above the minimum inhibitory concentration (MIC) during the dosing interval (t>MIC).
Clearance	Cefotaxime is partially metabolized by esterases in the liver and red blood cells. Desacetyl-cefotaxime is the major metabolite that has antibacterial activity and appears to work synergistically with the parent drug. Cefotaxime and its metabolites are **primarily excreted by the kidneys** through renal tubular secretion. Approximately 60% of an intravenous dose of cefotaxime is excreted unchanged and 24% as desacetyl-cefotaxime. The remainder are excreted as inactive metabolites. In older children, the **half-life of cefotaxime is approximately 1 hour** and the half-life of desacetyl-cefotaxime is 1.3 hours. The relatively short half-life makes frequent dosing necessary.

In neonates, the pharmacokinetics of cefotaxime is affected by gestational and chronological age. A longer half-life is seen in those born prematurely or with a low birth weight. In severe renal dysfunction the half-life of cefotaxime increases to approximately 2.5 hours and that of desacetyl-cefotaxime to approximately 10 hours. |

PRACTICAL PRESCRIBING

Dosing	The dose and frequency of administration are dependent on the age of the child, the severity and location of the infection and renal function. The standard recommended dose for children is **50 mg/kg three times a day**, increasing **to a maximum of four times a day in severe infections** and **suspected meningitis**. The **maximum daily dose is 12 g** even in those with severe infection. The dose is reduced and/or the frequency of administration **decreased when using cefotaxime in neonates** or those with renal impairment reflecting the prolonged half-life in these individuals. No dose adjustment is necessary for hepatic impairment.
Administration	Cefotaxime is only available as a parenteral formulation. It can be administered by IV bolus injection over 3–5 minutes, IV infusion over 20–60 minutes or deep IM injection. The powder should be reconstituted with sterile water for IV administration or **1% lignocaine for IM administration**.
Side effects and interactions	Severe allergic reactions and anaphylaxis are possible with cefotaxime so its use is contraindicated in individuals with a previous history of **immediate-type hypersensitivity to cephalosporins**. Due to cross-reactive allergy rates of 0.5–6.5% between penicillins and cephalosporins, the use of cefotaxime should be undertaken with **caution in penicillin-sensitive subjects**. It is probably best avoided if there has been a significant systemic reaction to penicillin. Other serious side effects include Stevens–Johnson syndrome, toxic epidermal necrolysis, haematological reactions and pseudomembranous colitis. As with other antibiotics, the prolonged use of cefotaxime may result in the bacterial overgrowth of non-susceptible organisms in the gut.
	Cefotaxime may **potentiate the nephrotoxic effects** of drugs such as **aminoglycosides and diuretics** such as furosemide so renal function should be monitored in these situations. Probenecid reduces the renal clearance of cefotaxime as it interferes with its renal tubular transfer. However, due to the large therapeutic index of cefotaxime, no dosage adjustment is needed unless renal function is impaired. Symptoms of overdose correspond to the recognized side effects. There is a risk of encephalopathy. In case of overdose, cefotaxime must be discontinued, and supportive treatment initiated. No specific antidote exists.
Monitoring	Routine monitoring of the cefotaxime plasma concentration is not necessary.
Cost	Cefotaxime is **relatively inexpensive**. A 500 mg ampoule costs around £2 and a 2 g ampoule costs around £4.

Ceftriaxone

CLINICAL PHARMACOLOGY

Why and when?	Ceftriaxone is a **third-generation cephalosporin antibiotic** (see Appendix 1 for more details of different generations of cephalosporins). It has a similar efficacy and safety profile to cefotaxime but its longer duration of action means it can be **given less frequently**. It is commonly used in hospital to treat children with proven or suspected septicaemia or **meningitis**. The **once-daily dosing regimen** is more convenient. In common with cefotaxime, it **has less activity against Gram-positive bacteria**, particularly *Staphylococcus aureus* than the second-generation cephalosporin cefuroxime.
Absorption and distribution	Ceftriaxone is poorly absorbed from the gastrointestinal tract and is converted to inactive metabolites by gut flora. It must **be given intravenously or intramuscularly**. It is distributed widely in tissues and fluids and achieves very similar peak serum levels to cefotaxime. At therapeutic plasma concentration plasma albumin binding is much higher than for cefotaxime, at around 85–95%.
Biology	Ceftriaxone is a **β-lactam antibiotic**, which is very similar to cefotaxime. Its structure means it is **resistant to the effects of β-lactamase**. Ceftriaxone exerts its **bactericidal** action by **inhibiting bacterial cell wall synthesis**. It binds to penicillin-binding proteins in the cell wall and inhibits peptidoglycan cross linkage. Ceftriaxone exhibits time-dependent killing.
Clearance	Ceftriaxone has an extended duration because ceftriaxone is **not significantly metabolized** and is **highly protein bound**. Unbound ceftriaxone is excreted unchanged in urine (60%) and bile (40%). The elimination half-life in older children is **around 8 hours**. This is prolonged in neonates and doses tend to be much lower in the first 2 weeks of life. In patients with either renal or hepatic impairment there is only a modest increase in elimination half-life as a reduction in one system of elimination is compensated by an increase in the other.

PRACTICAL PRESCRIBING

Dosing

	Neonate <15 d	**15–28 days old**	**1 m–11 yrs (<50kg)**	**>50 kg or >11 yrs**
Pneumonia, UTI, abdominal infection	20–50 mg/kg once daily (OD) IV	50–80 mg/kg OD IV	50–80 mg/kg OD (max 4 g) IV/IM	1–2 g OD (max 2 g) IV/IM
Skin, soft tissue, bone or joint infection	20–50 mg/kg OD IV	50–100 mg/kg OD IV	50–100 mg/kg OD (max 4 g) IV/IM	2 g OD IV/IM
Neutropenia with bacterial infection	20–50 mg/kg OD IV	50–100 mg/kg OD IV	50–100 mg/kg OD (max 4 g) IV/IM	2–4 g OD (max 4 g) IV/IM
Bacterial meningitis, endocarditis	50 mg/kg OD IV	80–100 mg/kg OD IV	80–100 mg/kg OD (max 4 g) IV/IM	2–4 g OD (max 4 g) IV/IM

Administration	Ceftriaxone can be administered IM or IV as a slow injection (over 5 min) or **preferably by infusion over 30–60 minutes**. For IV use the powder should be reconstituted in 5% glucose (10% in neonates) or 0.9% sodium chloride. If IM injection is required then the powder can be reconstituted in 1% lignocaine solution. **No more than 1 g should be given at any site and no more than 2 g in total should be delivered IM.**
Side effects and interactions	Severe **allergic reactions and anaphylaxis** are possible. It should not be given in individuals who report previous immediate-type hypersensitivity to cephalosporins. Similar to cefotaxime, the use of ceftriaxone should be undertaken with **caution in penicillin-sensitive subjects**. Other serious side effects include Stevens–Johnson syndrome, toxic epidermal necrolysis, haematological reactions and pseudomembranous colitis. The risk of less severe side effects such as diarrhoea, rash and elevated hepatic enzymes are more common than with cefotaxime. In neonates, ceftriaxone will **displace bilirubin from serum albumin** so cefotaxime is a better choice in jaundiced children.
	Ceftriaxone will bind calcium salts and this may result in precipitation, either in the vein or elsewhere (lungs, kidneys, liver and gallbladder). Due to these risks, ceftriaxone should not be reconstituted using a calcium-containing diluent and **calcium-containing infusions must not be administered via the same line as the ceftriaxone.** In overwhelming sepsis, where calcium can become rapidly depleted, this is an important consideration. Consider using cefotaxime in these circumstances. If used in resuscitation flush the line with 0.9% sodium chloride after administration.
Monitoring	Routine monitoring of plasma levels is not necessary. In children with severe renal and hepatic dysfunction, clinical monitoring for safety and efficacy is advised. It may potentiate the nephrotoxicity of drugs. Renal function should be monitored when used with aminoglycosides and diuretics.
Cost	Ceftriaxone is **fairly cheap,** costing about £10 per gram.

Cefuroxime

CLINICAL PHARMACOLOGY

Why and when?	Cefuroxime is a second-generation cephalosporin with a **broad antimicrobial activity** against both Gram-positive and Gram-negative organisms. It has excellent *in vitro* activity against staphylococcal strains, streptococcal strains (other than enterococci), *Neisseria gonorrhoeae*, *Haemophilus influenzae*, *Neisseria meningitides* and many Enterobacteriaceae. *Pseudomonas aeruginosa, Serratia marcescens* and some *Proteus species* are resistant.
	It distributes into bodily tissues and fluids, including the cerebrospinal fluid (CSF). The CSF penetration is unusual in second-generation cephalosporins. Cefuroxime is used successfully in the treatment of **pneumonia**, sepsis, **urinary tract**, **bone and joint**, skin, and soft tissue infections. It penetrates well into the intrapleural space and in higher doses is clinically effective in treatment of empyema. It is not used as first line for the treatment of bacterial meningitis as there is evidence that cefotaxime and ceftriaxone are more efficacious in *H. influenzae* meningitis.
Absorption and distribution	Cefuroxime comes in two forms, cefuroxime axetil for oral administration and sodium cefuroxime for parenteral use. Cefuroxime axetil is partially absorbed from the gastrointestinal tract, and this is **greater when taken after food** (bioavailability increases from 37% to 52%). Three-quarters of the cefuroxime dose is distributed in the extravascular compartment. Approximately **50%** of serum cefuroxime is **bound to protein**. It penetrates the placental barrier and is secreted during lactation.
Biology	Cephalosporins are **less susceptible to β-lactamases** than the penicillin β-lactam antibiotics. All β-lactams inhibit the formation of peptidoglycan cross-links within bacterial cell walls by targeting penicillin-binding proteins (PBPs). Consequently, the bacterial cell wall becomes weak and cytolysis occurs. It is usually **bactericidal**. Its precise structure means that it has a somewhat **broader range of activity** than the widely used third-generation cephalosporins, cefotaxime and ceftriaxone.
Clearance	Cefuroxime axetil is a **pro-drug**. After administration de-esterification occurs rapidly in the intestine, tissues and in blood to yield the **active form cefuroxime**. The axetil moiety is metabolized to acetaldehyde and acetic acid. Cefuroxime is metabolically stable, and most of it is excreted unchanged in the urine. The serum half-life after intravenous (IV) injection is just over 1 hour in adults but 3–5 times longer in neonates. Almost 90% of an IV dose of cefuroxime is renally excreted over 8 hours, resulting in **high urinary concentrations**. The half-life is prolonged in patients with renal impairment.

PRACTICAL PRESCRIBING

Dosing	Cefuroxime **dose is dependent** on the age of the child and location and **severity of infection**. Severe infections should be treated with IV cefuroxime and higher doses will somewhat increase the effectiveness and range of organisms treated. Dosing by mouth (for susceptible bacterial infections): Child 3 months–1 year: 10 mg/kg twice daily (max 125 mg per dose). Child 2–11 years: 15 mg/kg twice daily (max 250 mg per dose). Child 12–17 years: 250 mg twice daily, dose doubled in severe infection. By IV infusion, IV injection or intramuscular (IM) injection. For neonates IV only at 25 mg/kg 12 hourly in first 7 days of life, 8 hourly from 7–21 days and 6 hourly from 21–28 days. Doses doubled in severe infection. For children >1 month the dose is 20 mg/kg every 8 hours (max per dose 750 mg) **increased to 50–60 mg/kg** every 6–8 hours in **severe infections** and cystic fibrosis (max 1.5 g per dose).
Administration	Cefuroxime is available as an oral and parenteral formulation. Cefuroxime can be administered as **slow intravenous infusion**, IV injection or IM injection. The powder should be reconstituted in sterile water for IV administration or 1% lignocaine for IM administration. Single doses over 750 mg should be administered by the intravenous route only. For intermittent intravenous infusion, reconstituted solution should be diluted further in glucose 5% or sodium chloride 0.9% and given over 30 minutes.
Side effects and interactions	Cefuroxime is generally **well-tolerated** and its **side effects are usually transient**. If ingested after food, this antibiotic is both better absorbed and less likely to cause its most common side effects. Diarrhoea, nausea, vomiting, headaches/migraines, dizziness and abdominal pain are all seen at lower rates than most cephalosporins. It is contraindicated in patients with previous immediate hypersensitivity reaction to cephalosporins. Although a widely stated cross-allergic risk of about 10% exists between cephalosporins and penicillin, recent assessments have shown **no increased risk for a cross-allergic reaction for cefuroxime and several other second-generation or later cephalosporins**. The oral absorption of cefuroxime is diminished by reductions in gastric acid. Cefuroxime should be taken at least 1 hour before antacids are taken, or 2 hours afterwards. H_2-antagonists and proton pump inhibitors should be avoided during treatment with oral cefuroxime.
Monitoring	Routine monitoring of plasma concentration is not necessary.
Cost	Cefuroxime is **fairly cheap**. Gram for gram, 250 mg tablets are most expensive. Tablets cost between 35p (125 mg) and £1.25 (250 mg) each. Cefuroxime sodium powder for injection vials (250 mg and 750 mg) cost between £3-4 per gram. 70 mL of the oral suspension 125 mg/5 mL costs just over £5.

Chloral hydrate

CLINICAL PHARMACOLOGY

Why and when?	Chloral hydrate is a sedative and hypnotic. It has been used since the 1870s. In children it is mainly used to relieve anxiety and cause sedation before **non-invasive procedures and investigations**. Sometimes it is used as short-term management of **insomnia**. It induces quiet sleep. It is a relatively safe drug but may need to be monitored if higher doses are used because of risk of respiratory depression. It has **lower lethal therapeutic:toxic ratio** than diazepam.
Absorption	Main route of administration is oral. After oral or rectal administration, it is rapidly absorbed from the gastrointestinal tract with almost complete absorption. It undergoes extensive first-class metabolism in the liver producing an active metabolite called trichloroethanol. It is widely distributed. The estimated volume of distribution is 1–2 L/kg and 35–40% of trichloroethanol is bound to plasma proteins.
Biology	Chloral hydrate belongs to the class of organic compounds known as chlorhydrins. These are alcohols substituted by a chlorine atom at a saturated carbon atom otherwise bearing only hydrogen or hydrocarbyl groups. It is **metabolized by the liver and erythrocytes** to its active metabolite trichloroethanol. This reaction is catalysed primarily by alcohol dehydrogenase. Some of chloral hydrate and trichloroethanol is oxidized to trichloroacetic acid in the liver and kidneys. The precise **mechanism of action is unknown,** but chloral hydrate causes general **central nervous system (CNS) sedation** and induces quiet sleep but has no effect on REM sleep and has no analgesic properties. Trichloroethanol also undergoes glucuronidation to produce an inactive metabolite.
Clearance	Onset of action occurs **30–60 minutes** following enteral administration. Whilst the half-life of chloral hydrate itself is short, the half-life of its active metabolites are much longer (**8–12 hours for trichloroethanol**) which leads to a prolonged clinical effect of **4–8 hours**. The duration of action is subject to considerable inter-individual variability and can be up to 66 hours in neonates. Trichloroethanol, trichloroethanol glucuronide and trichloroacetic acid are excreted in the **urine**. Some trichloroethanol glucuronide may be secreted into bile and excreted in the faeces. Doses may need to be adjusted in cases of renal or hepatic impairment or alternative medicines should be used.

Triclofos or chloral hydrate?

Triclofos is the monophosphate sodium salt of trichloroethanol, the active metabolite of chloral hydrate. 1 g of triclofos sodium is broadly equivalent to 600 mg of chloral hydrate. Moreover, it is more palatable and produces less gastric irritation. However, this is not currently widely available in the UK.

Chloral hydrate

PRACTICAL PRESCRIBING

Dosing	Chloral hydrate is **given 45–60 minutes prior** to procedure or investigation. **Oral route is preferred but it can be given **rectally** if oral administration is not possible. For neonates and children <12 years of age, a dose of **30–50 mg/kg** (maximum 1 g) is given. If needed, doses of up to **100 mg/kg** (maximum 2 g) can be used under monitoring but there is a risk of respiratory depression. In children ≥12 years of age, a dose of **1–2 g** is used.
Administration	Chloral hydrate solution is unpalatable. The unpleasant taste makes administration difficult at times. It should be **diluted (1:3)** with water or juice before oral administration to mask its unpleasant taste. It should be **given with/following feeds** to decrease gastric irritation. Prolonged use of more than 2 weeks duration is not recommended. It is also available in tablet forms as chloral betaine. This is not as biologically active as the hydrate form, with 707 mg of chloral betaine being roughly equivalent to 414 mg of chloral hydrate.
Side effects and consideration	Chloral hydrate is a relatively safe drug and is generally well tolerated. Side effects include drowsiness, gastric and mucosal irritation, nausea, vomiting, diarrhoea, abdominal pain and headache. Higher doses can cause respiratory depression, myocardial depression, cardiac arrhythmias, vasodilation, hypotension and fluid retention. Drowsiness may persist the next day and affect performance of skilled tasks. It is contraindicated in severe cardiac disease, acute porphyrias and gastritis. It should not be used in severe renal or hepatic impairment. It should be used with caution in preterm neonates and in children with respiratory distress. It should be avoided in **pregnancy** as it can cause neonatal abstinence syndrome and in **breastfeeding** mothers. It should not be used in conjunction with other sedatives. Abrupt discontinuation can cause withdrawal symptoms. Prolonged use has been associated with hyperbilirubinemia, tolerance and physical dependence. **A patient information leaflet** is available at: https://www.medicines.org.uk/emc/product/8136/pil
Cost	Chloral hydrate solution is available as 143.3 mg/5 mL (28.66 mg/mL). It is **fairly expensive**, 1 g of oral solution costs approximately £57. It is also available as tablets, which contain 707 mg of chloral betaine, which is equivalent to 414 mg of chloral hydrate (pack of 30). Each tablet costs £4.60.

Chlorphenamine

CLINICAL PHARMACOLOGY

Why and when?	Chlorphenamine (also known as chlorpheniramine maleate) is a **first-generation antihistamine** and is most well known by its trade name Piriton®. It is used for **symptomatic relief of allergy** such as hay fever, allergic rhinitis, urticaria, food allergy, drug reactions. It is also used to **relieve itch** associated with chickenpox. It can be given orally, or if rapid onset of actions is required, e.g. **in anaphylaxis**, then it can be given parenterally (IV or IM).
Absorption and distribution	Oral doses of chlorphenamine are fairly well absorbed in the gastrointestinal tract. In adults the oral bioavailability of liquid and tablet formulations was 34% and 25%, respectively. There are small pharmacokinetic studies of oral dosing in children. These show that **absorption is usually rapid** but variable with peak plasma concentrations occurring at 1 hour in many children. The mean time to achieve peak concentrations following oral administration is 2.5 hours. Chlorphenamine is **highly lipid soluble** and therefore **crosses the blood–brain barrier** easily and leads to significant central nervous system effects. It is c.70% bound to plasma proteins in blood. It is considered as a **sedating antihistamine**.
Biology	Chlorphenamine is a potent histamine-1 receptor antagonist (**H_1-receptor antagonist**). It diminishes the actions of histamine in the body by **competitive reversible** blockade of H_1-receptor sites. It also has a small degree of anticholinergic (antimuscarinic) activity which explains some of its side effects. H_1 receptors are expressed widely. They are present in mast cells, smooth muscle, vascular endothelium, the heart and in the central nervous system. H_1-stimulation leads to vascular leak, bronchoconstriction and wakefulness, so blockade leads to **blockage of these effects**.
Clearance	Chlorphenamine is metabolized primarily in liver via cytochrome P450 (CYP450) enzymes. It has a fairly **prolonged duration of action**, which is longer still in adults and older children. The half-life is highly variable though at between 6 and 24 hours in children. Biological effects, i.e. blockade of wheal formation, persist for at least 24 hours and in children who have been taking regular chlorphenamine, for up to 3 days. Most antihistamines are present in breast milk in varying amounts but are not known to be harmful, but most manufacturers advise against their use in breastfeeding mothers.
Dosing	Whilst chlorphenamine is not licensed in children under 1 year of age, dosing schedules exist. In common with other antihistamines it appears relatively safe and has a **high therapeutic index**.

PRACTICAL PRESCRIBING

Dosing	For symptomatic relief of allergy then children under 2 (and older than 1 month) are given 1 mg twice a day initially. Children between 2 and 6 years are usually given 1 mg 4–6 hourly and can be given up to 6 mg/day. Children 6–12 years are given 2 mg 4–6 hourly up to a maximum of 12 mg per day and older children and adults are given 4 mg every 4–6 hours up to 24 mg per day. Doses for treatment of **anaphylaxis** are typically **much higher**, are given parenterally (**IV or IM**) and in younger children based on weight. Babies (<6 months old) require 250 micrograms/kg (max 2.5 mg) up to four times per day. Infants and young children (6 months–6 years) should have 2.5 mg up to four times in 24 hours. Older children (6–12 years) need 5 mg up to four times in 24 hours and adolescents and adults should have 10 mg up to four times in 24 hours.
Administration	There are oral suspensions and tablets available that can be brought as over-the-counter medicines for those over 1 year of age. **Oral suspensions are palatable** and children do not usually require encouragement to take them. Chlorphenamine for **injection can be given quickly**, i.e. by IV bolus over 1 minute. It can be diluted, if necessary, in 0.9% sodium chloride solution.
Side effects and interactions	**Drowsiness** is a significant side effect although paradoxical stimulation may occur, especially with high doses. It may diminish after a few days of regular treatment. Headache, motor impairment and antimuscarinic effects (urinary retention, dry mouth, blurred vision, constipation) all can occur in dose-dependent fashion. Rarer side effects include hypotension, palpitation, arrhythmias, extrapyramidal effects, dizziness, confusion, depression, sleep disturbances, tremor, convulsions, allergic reactions, blood disorders and liver dysfunction. Some over-the-counter cough and cold remedies contain chlorphenamine and care must be taken to avoid accidental overdose.
Monitoring	Routine monitoring of chlorphenamine plasma concentration is not necessary.
Cost	Oral solution and tablets are **cheap**. 4 mg tablets cost around 3p each and 150 mL of 2 mg/5 mL solution is only £2.21. Chlorphenamine injection is more expensive and a single vial of 10 mg/mL costs £4.50.

Ciclosporin

CLINICAL PHARMACOLOGY

Why and when?	Ciclosporin (cyclosporin) is a **calcineurin inhibitor**. It is a **potent immunosuppressant** used to suppress rejection in **organ transplant recipients** and to treat a variety of **chronic inflammatory and autoimmune diseases** including severe treatment-resistant **eczema** and **psoriasis** and **ulcerative colitis**. It also has a role in **nephrotic syndrome**. It is virtually non-myelotoxic but markedly nephrotoxic. Eye drops may be used for **severe vernal keratoconjunctivitis**.
Absorption and distribution	Oral formulations are mainly absorbed in the small intestine. Oral **absorption can be erratic and incomplete**. It is significantly dependent on presence of food, bile acids and gastrointestinal motility. **Food** taken at the same time will increase intestinal bile acid secretion and **enhances absorption**. Absorption is more variable in children than adults with factors like shorter bowel length and limited intestinal absorption being particularly important considerations.
	The **bioavailability** of oral solution in adults **is around 30%** and in children is **5–20%**. The time taken to peak in the serum is generally between 2 and 6 hours; but some patients may have a second peak at 5–6 hours. The reported volume of distribution of ciclosporin is high (4–8 L/kg). It tends to concentrate mainly on leucocyte-rich organs and in fatty tissues. Ciclosporin is lipophilic and crosses the blood–brain barrier although central nervous system levels are usually low as there are active efflux transport systems that oppose this.
Biology	Ciclosporin primarily **suppresses T cell cytokine production**. In particular it inhibits the transcription of the cytokine interleukin 2 (IL-2). It also inhibits the growth and activation of B cells and antigen-presenting cells, reduces the production of antibodies, inhibits degranulation and histamine release of mast cells, impairs leukotriene synthesis and downregulates the expression of adhesion molecules. Ciclosporin has some vasoconstrictor activities. In the kidneys, it has been shown to affect the proximal tubule and afferent arteriole, which may be one of the reasons that it is so **nephrotoxic** and can cause **hypertension**.
Clearance	Ciclosporin is almost completely eliminated **by hepatic metabolism**. The cytochrome P450 isoenzymes (e.g. CYP3A4) are important but there are more than 30 metabolites and several different systems are involved. Most of the metabolites are then eliminated in the bile. Its biological **half-life** is quite long and variable at about **18 hours** in adults but is generally shorter in children. Most cyclosporine metabolites (>90%) are **eliminated in the bile**. Clearance is then primarily via faeces.

PRACTICAL PRESCRIBING

Dosing	The dose regimen varies based on the condition and the degree of immunosuppression required. The usual initial oral dose is between **1 mg and 3 mg/kg twice daily** (depending upon indication). IV doses are usually between 0.5 mg and 1 mg/kg twice daily. The dose will be adjusted according to blood-ciclosporin concentration and clinical response. Doses are higher in organ transplant recipients. For keratoconjunctivitis, apply **1 drop 4 times a day**, to the affected eye(s). If signs and symptoms resolve then the dose is decreased to 1 drop twice daily.
Administration	In order to achieve stable blood levels it is important to give oral ciclosporin at the same time each day and around mealtimes. Mixing the solution with orange or apple juice improves palatability. Children should be stabilized on a **particular brand** of oral ciclosporin because switching between formulations may lead to clinically important changes in blood-ciclosporin concentration.
Side effects, errors and safety	Ciclosporin is **nephrotoxic**. Renal function must be checked **before initiation** and when used orally at regular intervals afterwards. It is an immunosuppressant and therefore children are at increased risk of serious infection. It also leads to **photosensitivity**, **excessive hair growth** (hypertrichosis) and **gum hypertrophy**. It can, rarely, lead to anaemia, thrombocytopenia and liver dysfunction and blood monitoring should include an intermittent full blood count and liver function test. Nausea, vomiting and headaches are all more common in the first few days after starting treatment but they usually wear off. Anaphylaxis has been reported with IV use. The Institute for Safe Medication Practices (ISMP) includes ciclosporin among its list of drugs that have a high risk of causing significant patient harm when used in error.
Monitoring	Ciclosporin concentrations reach steady state **only after 2–3 days**. Rapid dose alterations are not helpful. It is usual to change the dose by 10%, rounding off to the nearest 5 or 10 mg and not change the dose more than 20% at any single time. **Blood concentrations should not be measured until steady state is reached.** If a stable blood concentration changes suddenly, check for a new drug interaction before altering the dose; drugs that induce or inhibit CYP3A4 will significantly alter levels.
Cost	Ciclosporin is **moderately expensive**. 1 mL (100 mg/mL) of Neoral® oral solution costs just over £2 in the UK. 100 mg tablets or capsules also cost about £2 each, although there are small differences in the price between brands.

Ciprofloxacin

CLINICAL PHARMACOLOGY

Why and when?	Ciprofloxacin is a broad-spectrum antibiotic and belongs to the quinolone group of antibiotics. It is particularly active against Gram-negative bacteria but has some moderate activity against Gram-positive bacteria. Ciprofloxacin is used to treat *Salmonella*, *Shigella*, *Campylobacter*, *Neisseria* and *Pseudomonas aeruginosa*. It should not be used for pneumococcal pneumonia and has only moderate activity against *Streptococcus pneumoniae* and *Enterococcus faecalis*. It is active against *Chlamydia* and some mycobacteria. Ciprofloxacin is licensed in children over 1 year of age for **pseudomonal infections in cystic fibrosis**, complicated **urinary tract infection** and for treatment and prophylaxis of inhalation anthrax. It is also used for treatment of resistant **eye infections** and **otitis externa** that is resistant to initial treatment.
	When benefits outweigh the risk, **ciprofloxacin is licensed in children** over 1 year of age for severe respiratory tract, urinary tract and gastrointestinal infections (including Crohn's disease and typhoid fever). It is also used for treatment of septicaemia caused by multi-resistant organisms (usually hospital acquired) and gonorrhoea (resistance increasing). Ciprofloxacin is not licensed for the prophylaxis of meningococcal disease in children.
Absorption and distribution	Ciprofloxacin is **absorbed rapidly** from the gastrointestinal tract after oral administration and reaches peak plasma concentrations at about 2 hours. Bioavailability is high (c.70–80%) but is **reduced** by concomitant ingestion of **milk and fruit juice**. Around 20–40% is protein bound. Ciprofloxacin only poorly penetrates the blood–brain barrier.
Biology	The bactericidal action results from inhibition of the enzymes **topoisomerase II** (DNA gyrase) and **topoisomerase IV** (required for bacterial DNA replication, transcription, repair, strand supercoiling repair and recombination). This mechanism of action is different from that of other antimicrobial agents and there is no known cross-resistance; therefore, ciprofloxacin may be of use in organisms that are resistant to other antimicrobials. If used chronically, resistance can quickly emerge, particularly in *Pseudomonas aeruginosa* where there is activation of innate efflux mechanisms.
Clearance	Following ingestion it is metabolized in the liver. There is no substantial loss by first-pass metabolism. Approximately 40–50% of an orally administered dose is excreted in the urine as unchanged drug. Its **half-life is approximately 4 hours**.

PRACTICAL PRESCRIBING

Dosing	The dose and frequency of administration of ciprofloxacin are dependent on the age of the child, severity and source of infection. For respiratory infections in cystic fibrosis and severe respiratory, urinary tract or gastrointestinal infections in other children, the **oral dose** for children is **20 mg/kg (max 750 mg) twice daily** and the intravenous dose is 10 mg/kg (max 400 mg) 8-hourly. Neonates require lower doses. Doses should be adjusted in severe renal impairment.
Administration	Ciprofloxacin is one of the few broad-spectrum antibiotics available in both intravenous and oral formulations. **Eye drops** (3%) and **ointment** are available for superficial eye infections. **Ear drops** (2%) are available for treatment of otitis externa. Whilst tablets are cheaper, flavoured liquid formulations are available.
Contraindications, cautions and interactions	Quinolones cause **arthropathy** in the weight-bearing joints of immature animals and are therefore generally not recommended in children and growing adolescents. The significance of this effect in humans is uncertain and short-term use of ciprofloxacin may be justified in children. Ciprofloxacin is not licensed for children less than 1 year of age but neonatal dosing recommendations are given. Quinolone antibiotics may induce convulsions in patients with or without a history of convulsions. Taking non-steroidal anti-inflammatory drugs (NSAIDs) at the same time may also induce them.
	Tendon damage and rupture have been reported rarely and may occur within 48 hours of starting treatment. Cases have also been reported several months after stopping a quinolone. The risk of tendon damage is increased by the concomitant use of corticosteroids. **If tendonitis is suspected, the quinolone should be discontinued immediately**.
	Photosensitivity is relatively common and clinically important, particularly in children with cystic fibrosis who may receive oral ciprofloxacin in efforts to **eradicate newly acquired *Pseudomonas* infection.** Sun blocks should be advised and excessive exposure to sunlight should be avoided. Other common side effects are diarrhoea, dizziness, headache, nausea, vomiting.
Monitoring	Routine monitoring of levels or other blood parameters is not necessary.
Cost	The cost is dependent on formulation used. **Tablets are very cheap** (currently the lowest cost 500 mg tablet is around £8 for 100). Eye drops and ear drops are fairly inexpensive (£4–5 for a treatment course) but the **oral suspension is relatively expensive** (around £21 for 100 mL of oral suspension). As the oral bioavailability is good, intravenous treatment is rarely needed but a single 400 mg dose costs around £10.

Clarithromycin

CLINICAL PHARMACOLOGY

Why and when?	Clarithromycin is a **macrolide antibiotic**. Other examples include erythromycin and azithromycin. Clarithromycin has some advantages over erythromycin including **fewer side effects**, better bioavailability, longer half-life and wider antimicrobial coverage. It is recommended for the treatment of **community-acquired pneumonia** and can be used safely in children with **penicillin allergy**. It is also used for skin and soft-tissue infections, otitis media, sinusitis and prevention of pertussis. Less commonly it is used for treatment of Lyme disease in penicillin-allergic children and in treatment of *Helicobacter pylori* infection as part of several triple-drug therapy regimens.
Absorption and distribution	Clarithromycin is stable in acidic medium and is **well absorbed from the gastrointestinal tract**, regardless of the presence of food. After an oral dose about 50% of the dose is absorbed in healthy adults and oral clarithromycin reaches peak serum concentrations within 2 hours. Oral bioavailability is about double that of erythromycin. There are few advantages to the intravenous preparations, which are irritant to veins. Both clarithromycin and the 14-OH metabolite distribute widely into body tissues and fluids. Levels in lung epithelial lining fluid reach concentrations **15–20 times higher than plasma concentrations**. Levels in lung alveolar macrophages are typically >200 times higher than serum levels. There are no data on cerebrospinal fluid (CSF) penetration.
Biology	Like other macrolides, clarithromycin exerts its antibacterial action **by binding to the 50S ribosomal subunit of susceptible organisms**, thereby blocking RNA-mediated bacterial protein synthesis and inhibiting bacterial growth. Clarithromycin can be bacteriostatic or bactericidal in action, depending on the concentration achieved and the target organism. Clarithromycin has demonstrated bactericidal activity against both typical and atypical respiratory pathogens. It has good activity against group A streptococcus, *Streptococcus pneumoniae*, *Moraxella catarrhalis*, *Mycoplasma pneumoniae*, *Bordetella pertussis*, *Legionella pneumophila*, *Chlamydia pneumoniae*, *Chlamydia trachomatis*, *Neisseria gonorrhoeae*, *Helicobacter pylori* and *Propionibacterium acnes*. It has been found to be not very active against methicillin-resistant *Staphylococcus aureus*, coagulase-negative staphylococci and enterococci.
Clearance	Once absorbed, clarithromycin is significantly (65–75%) protein bound. Clarithromycin is primarily metabolized in the liver by cytochrome P450 CYP3A isozymes and has an active metabolite, 14-hydroxyclarithromycin. It has a relatively long **half-life of approximately 3 hours**, which permits twice daily dosing. Clarithromycin is eliminated by both renal and hepatic mechanisms. About 20–40% is excreted in the urine as unchanged drug; additional 10–15% as a metabolite. In faeces 29–40% is excreted mostly as metabolite.

PRACTICAL PRESCRIBING

Dosing	For respiratory tract (including otitis media/sinusitis), skin and soft tissue infection babies <8 kg should receive 7.5 mg/kg twice daily orally or intravenously. Heavier children usually have **weight-banded doses for oral treatment:** 8–11 kg infants require 62.5 mg, 12–19 kg children need 125 mg, 20–30 kg children 187.5 mg and heavier children have 250 mg, all twice daily. Doses in children over 12 years can be doubled in severe infection. If used intravenously the dose is usually 7.5 mg/kg with a maximum dose of 500 mg, again twice daily. **It is highly irritant to the veins** and whenever possible a large vein or central line should be used. IV clarithromycin should not be used for more than 5 days.
Administration	Oral clarithromycin comes either in the immediate-release preparation or modified-release preparation. **The immediate-release preparation is mainly used in paediatrics**. It comes in granules, tablets and oral suspension. The immediate-release tablet formulations and oral suspensions can be taken with or without food whereas the clarithromycin extended-release tablets should be administered with food. Tablets and the IV infusion are not licensed for use in children <12 years, oral suspension is not licensed for use in infants <6 months.
Side effects	Clarithromycin is relatively well tolerated. It has a strong bitter taste and some children will still not take liquid suspensions. In palatability tests there is **significant variation between the different available paediatric brands** and sometimes a child will take one brand when another is refused. Granules can be helpful but are often difficult to source. The main side effect of clarithromycin is gastrointestinal upset (vomiting, diarrhoea and abdominal pain); however, these are uncommon and occur in about 7% of patients. Other side effects include taste disturbances, headache, and QT prolongation if used with inhaled anaesthetics, clotrimazole, antiarrhythmic agents, or azoles. Clarithromycin should be used cautiously in patients with renal insufficiency or liver failure. It has a similar drug interaction profile to erythromycin and has been reported to potentiate the effect of astemizole, carbimazole, corticosteroids, cyclosporine, digoxin, ergot alkaloids and theophylline.
Cost	Clarithromycin is **cheaper than azithromycin but more expensive than erythromycin**. Its cost depends on the formulation/concentration. The oral suspension 25 mg/mL costs about £3.12 for a 70 mL bottle and the 50 mg/1 mL suspension costs about £3.84 for a 70 mL bottle. 250 mg tablets cost £1.18 for 14 tablets, 500 mg tablets cost about £1.87 for 14 tablets and modified-release 500 mg tablets cost £13.23 for 14 tablets. 500 mg powder for concentration for solutions of infusion vials cost £9.45 per vial and the 250 mg granules sachet costs £11.68 for 14 sachets.

Clobazam

CLINICAL PHARMACOLOGY

Why and when?	Clobazam has been widely used for years and has been proven effective as an **adjunctive therapy in primary generalized and partial epilepsy**. It is a useful 'add-on' treatment in tonic–clonic, complex partial, myoclonic seizures and in the treatment of seizures associated with **Lennox–Gastaut syndrome**. Clobazam can also be used as monotherapy for non-refractory focal and generalized childhood epilepsies. It is sometimes used in short courses to cover increasing clusters of seizures and has a particular indication for catamenial (menstruation) seizures. The effectiveness of clobazam may decrease significantly after weeks or months of continuous therapy due to **tolerance** developing.
Absorption	Clobazam is well absorbed from the gut, and its lipid solubility ensures ready penetration into the brain. Tablet and oral suspension have an **oral bioavailability of >95%**. It has a **rapid onset** (30 minutes–4 hours) and an **extended duration** of action. Oral suspension forms are slightly more rapidly absorbed and may therefore have a quicker onset of action. It belongs to the long-acting (>24 hours) benzodiazepines. Taking the medication with food does not significantly affect absorption.
Biology	The mechanism of action for clobazam is not fully understood but is thought to involve what is known as **potentiation of GABAergic neurotransmission**, resulting from binding at a benzodiazepine site at the $GABA_A$ receptor. It ends to produce **less sedation than other benzodiazepines**, perhaps because it has lower affinity for the ω_1 site of the $GABA_A$ receptor.
Clearance	Once absorbed most clobazam is protein bound (80–90%). Its **half-life is relatively long** and ranges from 20 to 40 hours. Clobazam is converted to N-desmethylclobazam, a partially active metabolite in the liver by CYP450 enzymes including CYP3A4 and CYP2C19 enzymes. N-desmethylclobazam has a longer half-life (about 80 hours) and approximately 20% of the biological activity of clobazam. Due to its extended half-life, N-desmethylclobazam may begin to accumulate after prolonged use. Some other antiepileptic drugs (carbamazepine, phenobarbital and phenytoin) are CYP3A4 inducers. Both clobazam and N-desmethylclobazam are then predominantly (>90%) renally excreted.

Giving children suspension formulations of drugs

There are some important practical steps to take when giving children medicines in suspension form. For some drugs, including clobazam, it is important to shake the bottle before use and also to use a syringe or medicine spoon to reduce the risk of dosing errors. Using household teaspoons (or tablespoons) results in very variable volumes and should be discouraged.

PRACTICAL PRESCRIBING

Dosing	Oral clobazam suspension is available in the strength 10 mg/5 mL and 5 mg/5 mL. Tablets are available as 10 mg. It is most often used as an adjunct therapy in epilepsy. **Dosing is age- and weight-dependent**.

The dosing for most indications in children aged 1 month-5 years is initially 125 microgram/kg twice daily. The dose is then increased, if necessary every 5 days to a maintenance dose of 250 microgram/kg twice daily (maximum dose of 500 microgram/kg twice daily or 30 mg per day).

In children 6–17 years the initial dose is 5 mg daily, increased, if necessary, at intervals of 5 days to a maintenance dose of 0.3–1 mg/kg daily. Daily doses of up to 30 mg may be given as a single dose at bedtime, with higher doses being divided, with a maximum 60 mg per day. |
| Side effects and considerations | Common side effects in children include **drowsiness**, decreased energy and difficulties with coordination or balance. Children may also become aggressive or easily irritated. These effects often improve after about a week from starting the medication. A few children get a mild tremor of their fingers that usually gets better after a few weeks. A drug-related skin rash is very rare. Clobazam will have **increased oral and respiratory secretions**, which can be a particular problem in children with significant neurodisability.

An important concern when people with epilepsy take clobazam is that **seizures will become more frequent or more severe if the medicine is lowered or stopped**. The longer the person has been taking clobazam and the higher the dose, the greater the tolerance and therefore the higher the risk of worsening seizure control. Therefore small and gradual dose reductions over a number of months are necessary. |
| Monitoring | All infants and children taking clobazam should be monitored for sedation, feeding difficulties, adequate weight gain and developmental milestones. No therapeutic drug monitoring is routinely recommended. |
| Cost | Clobazam oral suspension is **moderately expensive** with a 150 mL bottle costing around £80–100, these need to be ordered ahead by pharmacies. 10 mg tablets are cheaper costing £3.65 for a pack of 30 tablets. |

Codeine phosphate

CLINICAL PHARMACOLOGY

Why and when?	Codeine is classed as a **weak opioid analgesic**, with a quick onset of action. It is used primarily as analgesia; however, it also has sedative, hypnotic, anti-nociceptive and anti-peristaltic effects. Its analgesic qualities are brought about by the conversion of codeine to morphine when taken. Codeine was widely used in children until recently when case reports emerged of **unexpected respiratory depression in children** following surgery. This has led to a significant reduction in use.
Absorption and distribution	Codeine is usually **administered orally**. Oral codeine has a **rapid onset of action** of 10–15 minutes and a likely **bioavailability of c.50% in humans**. The clinical effects peak at between 30 minutes and 1 hour and clinical **effects last up to 4–6 hours** with shorter durations of action in younger children. When taken regularly, a steady state of codeine can be achieved but the half-life is difficult to predict due to **variations in codeine metabolism** (see Clearance below). Codeine can also be administered parenterally but this is rarely done due the risk of an anaphylactoid response.
Biology	Codeine is a **weak opioid analgesic**. Codeine itself is a selective agonist for the μ-opioid receptor, but with a much weaker affinity to this receptor than morphine. Most of the analgesic properties of codeine are thought to arise from its **conversion to morphine** by the cytochrome P450 enzyme **CYP2D6**. It has an observed potency of about 1/10th of that seen for morphine which correlates reasonably well with its *in vivo* conversion to morphine (c.5–15% – see Clearance below).
Clearance	Codeine is eliminated either by direct renal excretion (5–15% is found unchanged in the urine) or following **hepatic metabolism**. In the liver most codeine (c.50–70%) undergoes **glucuronidation to codeine-6-glucuronide**, an inactive metabolite **or N-demethylation to norcodeine** (c.10–20%). However, c.5–15% will undergo **O-demethylation to morphine**. The half-life and, in particular, the clinical effects of codeine are highly variable due to genetic variation in CYP2D6.

Pharmacogenomics and CYP2D6 genotype

In Caucasian populations 1–2% of children are 'ultra-rapid' metabolizers who have more than two functional 'wild-type' alleles and 5–10% of children are poor metabolizers (no functional alleles). Ultra-fast metabolizers will rapidly convert codeine to morphine and are at significant increased risk from standard codeine doses. Unfortunately, in clinical practice it is rare to know in advance whether a child will be an ultra-fast metabolizer (at increased risk of unanticipated toxicity) or a poor metabolizer (who will find codeine is a poor analgesic).

PRACTICAL PRESCRIBING

Dosing	Codeine is **no longer recommended for any child under the age of 12 years.** This is due to the increased risk of respiratory depression, especially neonates. For the treatment of pain, codeine is usually given by the oral route. For children and young people over 12 years the dose is 30–60 mg 3–4 times a day. The maximum daily dose is 240 mg a day in divided doses, but it should only be used for short-term treatment, i.e. a maximum of 72 hours. For acute diarrhoea the usual dose is 15–60 mg 3–4 times daily; again, this is indicated in children over 12 years of age.
Administration	Codeine can be given by the **oral or rectal** routes. Much less commonly it is given via the IM route. The bioavailability of IM codeine is probably around 70% and dose reductions may be required.
Side effects and considerations for use	General side effects of all opioids include hypotension, confusion, constipation, drowsiness, dry mouth, euphoria, hallucinations, headache, nausea, palpitations, skin reactions and urinary retention. **Care must be given when codeine is first administered as the biological effects may be variable**. If a child is sent home on codeine, parents must be aware of the common side effects and what to look out for. A helpful information leaflet for parents is available at https://www.medicinesforchildren.org.uk/codeine-phosphate-pain-0. If there are signs of toxicity (e.g. respiratory depression, unconsciousness, constricted pupils), then an antidote should be administered in hospital. Naloxone, which competitively binds μ-opioid receptors, is effective in overdose.
Monitoring	Drug levels are not routinely monitored but **children should have a set of clinical observations taken 30 minutes after the first dose** of codeine to check for respiratory depression or other toxic effects.
Cost	Oral codeine **is inexpensive**, one 30 mg tablet costs 2–3p; however, this can vary depending on the brand. Oral solution is slightly more expensive at around 10p per 30 mg dose. For IM administration 1 ampoule of 60 mg costs £2.41. Codeine suppositories are not widely available in the UK.

Colomycin

CLINICAL PHARMACOLOGY

Why and when?	Colomycin is used for the treatment of **Gram-negative organisms**, particularly ***Pseudomonas aeruginosa*** but also *Acinetobacter baumannii* and *Klebsiella pneumoniae*. It can be given intravenously, via inhaled powder or in a nebulized form. Colomycin nebulizers are used in the management of chronic *P. aeruginosa* infection in patients with cystic fibrosis. Inhaled powder can be used as an alternative to nebulizers if they are not tolerated. It is usually bactericidal. Colomycin (colistimethate sodium) is an inactive prodrug of colistin. It is not stable *in vivo* and is hydrolyzed in human plasma, creating a mixture of derivatives including colistin.
Absorption and distribution	Colomycin is **not absorbed orally**. Distribution in lung parenchyma, pericardial and pleural fluid and cerebrospinal fluid is poor. However, clinical studies have shown that the vast majority of lung pathogenic bacteria (i.e. *P. aeruginosa*) are located within the mucus/sputum, therefore clinical efficacy of inhaled or nebulized therapies is good. Following intravenous (IV) administration peak plasma levels of colistin are achieved rapidly (<10 minutes).
Biology	Colomycin is a polymyxin antibiotic. It works by binding to lipopolysaccharides and phospholipids on the **outer membrane of gram-negative bacteria**. It competitively displaces calcium and magnesium from phosphate groups of membrane lipids. This leads to **disruption of the outer cell membrane**, leakage of intracellular contents and bacterial death. The **extracellular site of action** reduces the ability of organisms to develop resistance, even when used continuously.
Clearance	Colomycin is renally excreted. However, *in vivo* it is converted to its active form, colistin, and the mechanism of excretion of colistin is unclear. The **half-life** in healthy individuals and those with cystic fibrosis is **usually 2–3 hours**. Although the precise elimination route is unclear, dose reductions are recommended for patients with creatinine clearance <50 mL/minute.

Colomycin and drug resistance

Colomycin is one of the few critical antibacterial drugs for treating multidrug-resistant bacteria and is listed on the WHO Essential Medicines List (EML) as a last-resort antibiotic.

Colomycin-resistance has been slow to emerge due to its extracellular mechanism of action. When it does occur it has mostly been due to non-transmissible chromosomal mutations. However, a transmissible colistin resistance gene (*mcr*) was reported in 2015. This raises the possibility of rapid transfer of colomycin-resistance to other bacterial species and is being carefully monitored.

In clinical practice, *in vivo* resistance is uncommon but does often emerge in older children and adults with prolonged *P. aeruginosa* infection.

PRACTICAL PRESCRIBING

Dosing	For IV administration: Children with body weight up to 41 kg: 75,000–150,000 units/kg daily divided into 3 doses. Children 41 kg or over: 9 million units should be given daily divided into 2–3 doses. For nebulized administration: Children 1–23 months: 0.5–1 million units twice daily. Children >2 yrs: 1–2 million units 2–3 times a day. For inhalation of powder: 1.66 million units twice daily.
Administration	Colomycin can be administered intravenously, via nebulizer or as an inhaled powder. Doses are typically given 2–3 times per day. Whilst powder formulations are typically more expensive, they can be delivered more rapidly which **may improve adherence**.
Side effects and interactions	Colomycin is known to reduce the presynaptic release of acetylcholine at the neuromuscular junction and should not be used in patients with myasthenia gravis. Commoner side effects when nebulized include bronchospasm, cough, chest discomfort, dyspnoea, altered taste, vomiting, throat problems and tinnitus. Side effects for IV administration are rare but include confusion, **nephrotoxicity**, pre-syncope, psychosis, neurological issues including neurotoxicity and apnoea. Nephrotoxic and neurotoxic **side effects are dose related**. No medications are absolutely contraindicated when used concurrently with colomycin. However, there are numerous medications that when used with colomycin (particularly IV) increase risk of nephrotoxicity; these include diclofenac, ibuprofen, amikacin, amphotericin, cefotaxime, ceftazidime, ciclosporin, tacrolimus, trimethoprim and many more. Medications with neuromuscular blocking effects, such as amikacin, gentamicin and neomycin, should also be used with caution.
Monitoring	With IV use, renal function should be monitored. With inhaled use, lung function should be performed before and after the first dose and the patient **should be monitored for bronchospasm**. Should bronchospasm occur, the test should be repeated with a bronchodilator.
Cost	Colomycin is a **fairly expensive antibiotic**. A single 1 million-unit vial for injection costs £1.80 and a 2 million-unit vial costs £3.24. A single million-unit vial for nebulizer costs £6.80 and inhaled powder is even more expensive with a 1.66 million-unit vial costing £17.30. Annual treatment cost for powder is £12,629 per individual.

Desmopressin

CLINICAL PHARMACOLOGY

Why and when?	Desmopressin is an analogue of vasopressin (also known as antidiuretic hormone (ADH)). Desmopressin has several indications. It is used as a treatment in primary **nocturnal enuresis**, usually after a trial of non-pharmacological treatment, and is also used in the treatment of **diabetes insipidus**. In mild to moderate **haemophilia** and **von Willebrand's disease** it is used to increase plasma concentration of factor VIII and von Willebrand factor during episodes of bleeding or for procedures.
Absorption and distribution	Absorption varies dependent upon the route of administration. Desmopressin in **oral form** has a **relatively low bioavailability**, typically it is approximately 0.1% in adult studies and therefore there is a big difference in the amount required orally and intravenously. The sublingual form is typically more bioavailable and 120 micrograms (mcg) of the sublingual dose is roughly equivalent to 200 mcg of the oral form. The bioavailability of intranasal doses is approximately 20% and 20–25 times lower doses are required to achieve similar effects. It does not cross the blood–brain barrier. Peak plasma levels are reached 30–60 minutes after intravenous (IV) dosing, 60–90 min after intranasal administration and 1–2 hours after oral or sublingual dosing. The time of **peak effect** depends upon the desired action, **effects on nocturia** occur within **15–45 min**, whereas peak effects on **factor VIII** and von Willebrand factor occur within **30–90 min**.
Biology	Desmopressin is more potent and has a longer duration of action than vasopressin. Unlike vasopressin, desmopressin has no vasoconstrictor effect.
	Desmopressin acts selectively on the vasopressin type-2 (V2) receptor. In the context of nocturnal **enuresis** and **diabetes insipidus**, desmopressin works by **mimicking the actions of vasopressin** in the **kidney**. It increases the reabsorption of water by increasing the water permeability of the cortical and medullary **collecting tubules**, meaning a smaller volume of more concentrated urine is produced. Whereas it stimulates the **production of factor VIII** and **von Willebrand factor** from **endothelial cells,** also by acting upon V2 receptors. Desmopressin leads to a two-fold to 20-fold increase in the plasma concentration of factor VII.
Clearance	The drug is substantially **excreted by the kidney** and so the risk of toxicity may increase in the presence of renal impairment. The hormone vasopressin has a half-life of around 10 minutes and a short duration of action; however, desmopressin is subject to less degradation by tissue peptidases so has a plasma **half-life of approximately 75 min**. Oral doses take longer to reach peak concentration and have a longer biological half-life of **1.5–2.5 hours**. There is considerable **circadian variation** in the pharmacokinetic parameters of desmopressin. In studies involving adults, the half-life is **longer at night** than during the day.

PRACTICAL PRESCRIBING

Dosing	Dosing is variable depending on age, indication and route of administration. For children over 12 years with diabetes insipidus the starting dose is 100 mcg three times a day orally. The maintenance dose is variable and usually between 200 mcg and 1.2 mg per day. Younger children need lower doses. For **nocturnal enuresis** children over 5 years are usually commenced on 200 mcg orally or 120 mcg sublingually. If this is ineffective then a double dose can be tried. The **intranasal dose** for haemophilia or von Willebrand's disease in children aged 1–17 years is 4 mcg/kg (max 300 mg), given 2 hours before procedure when used pre-operatively. As bioavailability is 20% by this route it delivers a much higher dose than oral forms. If IV desmopressin is given, doses are far lower.
Administration	Desmopressin is available for administration by oral, sublingual, intranasal, subcutaneous, intramuscular or IV routes. In the tablet form there are 100- and 200 mcg doses, with a 200 mcg desmotab available, and solution for oral use has one strength of 360 mcg per 1 mL. Lysophilate oral melts for sublingual use have 60-, 120- and 240 mcg dosages. For **nocturnal enuresis** the nasal route is not recommended due to the risk of increased side effects. It is also advised that children should **not have anything to drink** for **1 hour before** they take desmopressin, and then for **8 hours after** they have taken it.
Side effects and interactions	Common side effects include **hyponatraemia**, when administered without restricting fluid intake, and nausea. It also may cause mild headaches and stomach pain. These often get better after a few days. Very rarely, a child may become more aggressive when taking desmopressin.

It is contraindicated in patients with cardiac insufficiency, treated with diuretics, a history of hyponatraemia or polydipsia. Lamotrigine and chlorpromazine increase the risk of hyponatraemia. Loperamide greatly increases the absorption of oral forms. |
| Monitoring | Fluid input must be managed carefully to avoid hyponatraemia, and serum electrolytes may need to be monitored. Rarely, desmopressin can lead to hyponatraemic convulsions. Signs of fluid retention should prompt reassessment of dosage and suitability. **After 3 months** of treatment for nocturnal enuresis then a **withdrawal of treatment for 1 week** is recommended to see if it is still required. |
| Cost | Oral desmopressin is **fairly cheap** but cost varies depending on the medicinal form. The cheapest oral dose is currently around £0.35 per dose (£10.56 for 30 tablets). Branded oral and sublingual forms are costlier (about £1 per dose). Solution for injection costs c.£13 for 10 ampoules of 4 mcg/mL. |

Dexamethasone

CLINICAL PHARMACOLOGY

Why and when?

Dexamethasone is a synthetic glucocorticoid. It has anti-inflammatory and immunosuppressive effects. It is commonly used in the **treatment of croup** and for **cerebral oedema** as well as for **physiological replacement** in glucocorticoid insufficiency. It is often used prior to extubation if there is minimal or no leak around the endotracheal tube. Dexamethasone is known to reduce the risk of hearing loss and neurological complications in **bacterial meningitis**. It also has an **antiemetic** effect although it is less commonly used for this effect. Dexamethasone has a well-established safety and efficacy profile in all ages. Dexamethasone is available in oral, intravenous (IV) and intramuscular (IM) forms as well as in an eye drop form.

Absorption

Oral dexamethasone has a **high bioavailability** (60–85%). Studies in adults with gastric stasis suggest that it is absorbed readily from the stomach. The time to peak serum concentration is **rapid** and approximately **1–2 hours** for both oral and IV dexamethasone. Dexamethasone rapidly crosses the blood–brain barrier.

Biology

Dexamethasone is a **glucocorticoid agonist** with **little or no mineralocorticoid effects**. It acts to modify protein synthesis in order to reduce the production of inflammatory mediators and suppressing neutrophil migration thus suppressing a normal immune response and reducing inflammation. This process involves phospholipase A2 inhibitory proteins, which control the production of prostaglandins and leukotrienes. Dexamethasone also has an antiemetic effect but the mechanism of this is not known.

Clearance

Dexamethasone is primarily **metabolized in the liver.** It is broken down to inactive glucuronide and sulfate metabolites. These inactive metabolites and small amounts of unmetabolized dexamethasone are **excreted by the kidneys**. The biological half-life for dexamethasone varies with age but in general is fairly long. The relatively long half-life leads to a **fairly prolonged clinical effect even from a single dose**. For a neonate the half-life is between 5 and 16 hours and for children aged 4 months to 16 years it is between 36 and 54 hours. Certain drugs (e.g. phenobarbital, phenytoin and rifampicin) increase the metabolism of glucocorticoids by increasing activity of GYP3A4.

Palatability of oral steroids

Experience and observational studies suggest that oral dexamethasone liquid is palatable. This is an important consideration, particularly if the child has airway compromise and may get upset by an unpleasant medicine. Children prefer it to oral prednisolone and it is less likely to lead to nausea or vomiting. If a child does vomit within 30 minutes of dexamethasone dosing it should be repeated.

PRACTICAL PRESCRIBING

Dosing	Dexamethasone dosing is primarily **weight-based**. Dosing for physiological replacement is based on surface area, 250–500 micrograms (mcg)/m^2 should be given every 12 hours.

Dosing for suppression of inflammation or allergic reaction is 10–100 mcg/kg/day orally in divided doses, 300 mcg/kg/day may be used in emergencies. For IM and IV dosing the range is 83–333 mcg/kg/day in divided doses to a maximum of 20 mg daily.

In **croup** the initial dose is usually **150 mcg/kg orally**, which can be repeated after 12 hours if needed. The onset of action in croup is **very fast**. Clinical effects are seen within 30 minutes but it may take 4 hours to have maximal effect. In **bacterial meningitis** the dose is also **150 mcg/kg** but it is given 6-hourly. In life-threatening cerebral oedema the dose is much higher. Children weighing up to 35 kg should have 16.7 mg initially and then 3.3 mg every 3 hours for 3 days and then wean. For children >35 kg then 20.8 mg should be given initially then 3.3 mg 2-hourly for 3 days and then wean. |
| Administration | Oral dexamethasone is available is both **tablet and liquid** forms. Soluble tablets should be dispersed in water. Non-soluble tablets can, if necessary, be crushed and mixed with yoghurt, honey or jam. However, chewing should be discouraged. Oral dexamethasone is also available in 2 mg/5 mL, 10 mg/5 mL and 20 mg/5 mL liquid solution. |
| Drug errors and safety | Long-term use of systemic dexamethasone can lead to side effects. It can cause **immunosuppression** and increase susceptibility to infections. In particular children who are not immune to chickenpox are at risk of developing **severe chickenpox** and should, whenever possible, avoid exposure to the virus. Dexamethasone can also affect **mood and behaviour**, rarely causing steroid-induced psychosis. It can cause gastric irritation for which proton-pump inhibitor cover is commonly co-prescribed.

If any systemic steroid has been given for **more than 21 days** then it is necessary to gradually **wean** dosing until it is stopped. Moreover, children taking long-term glucocorticoids (including dexamethasone) who become acutely unwell will need additional glucocorticoid cover and typically the regular dose is doubled during the illness.

Due to the above potential risks, children who are prescribed this drug on a long-term basis should be given a steroid card that contains their medication details. |
| Monitoring | Children receiving long-term treatment with dexamethasone require **serial height and weight monitoring:** firstly to ensure dosing is adjusted to growth and secondly to monitor growth. |
| Cost | Dexamethasone is **cheap**. The solution for injection costs £2.02 for a 3.3 g/1 mL ampoule of dexamethasone. This is more expensive than the oral forms, which cost £0.60 per 2 mg soluble tablet, £0.28 per 2 mg non-soluble tablet and £1.44 for 2 mg of oral suspension. |

Digoxin

CLINICAL PHARMACOLOGY

Why and when?	Digoxin is a **cardiac glycoside** derived from the *Digitalis* (foxglove) plant. It **increases the contractility of the heart** and is used to treat **heart failure**. Digoxin is usually indicated in cases of heart failure with persistent symptoms despite treatment with other agents (i.e. diuretics, ACE inhibitors). It also **reduces the heart rate** and is useful in the treatment of supraventricular tachyarrhythmias.
Absorption and distribution	Digoxin is **well absorbed** from the gastrointestinal tract with a bioavailability of 60–70%. It has a **large volume of distribution** because it accumulates in the peripheral tissues and especially the muscles. The distribution phase is typically long and lasts 6–8 hours. Its pharmacologic effects are **delayed** and do not correlate well with serum concentrations during the distribution phase. Neonates, infants and young children have significantly larger volumes of distribution than older children and adults. The protein-bound fraction of the drug is 25%.
Biology	Digoxin is an inotropic agent. It **inhibits the Na^+/K^+-ATPase** pump in myocardial cells resulting in a transient increase of intracellular sodium, which in turn promotes **calcium influx** via the sodium–calcium exchange pump leading to **increased contractility**. Digoxin also directly suppresses the atrioventricular (AV) node conduction to **increase effective refractory period** and decrease conduction velocity. Thus, it can **decrease the heart rate in atrial tachyarrhythmias**.
Clearance	Digoxin is mainly excreted **unchanged in the urine**. A small proportion of the drug (c.16%) is metabolized. The metabolites may contribute to the therapeutic and toxic effects. Digoxin has typically a **long half-life**; 35–45 hours in term neonates, 18–25 hours in infants and 18–36 hours in children. In preterm neonates the half-life is very prolonged (61–170 hours). Renal impairment decreases clearance and prolongs half-life.
Dosing	The dose of administration is dependent on the age and weight of the child, the condition and the renal function. **Infants and young children** have larger volumes of distribution and clearance than older children and adults and therefore **require higher doses per kg**. Digoxin treatment is initiated with a **loading** (digitalizing) dose that is administered in 3 divided doses over 24 hours. This is followed by a **maintenance dose** that is given once or twice daily. Doses may need to be reduced if a child has received digoxin in the last 2 weeks. Dose reductions are necessary in renal impairment.

PRACTICAL PRESCRIBING

Age group		Total loading dose (in 3 divided doses over 24 hours)	Total daily maintenance dose (in 1–2 divided doses)
Neonate	Weight <1.5 kg	PO: 25 mcg/kg IV: 20 mcg/kg	PO: 4–6 mcg/kg IV: 4–6 mcg/kg
	1.5–2.5 kg	PO: 30 mcg/kg IV: 30 mcg/kg	PO: 4–6 mcg/kg IV: 4–6 mcg/kg
	>2.6 kg	PO: 45 mcg/kg IV: 35 mcg/kg	PO: 10 mcg/kg IV: 10 mcg/kg
Child	1 month–1 year	PO: 45 mcg/kg IV: 35 mcg/kg	PO: 10 mcg/kg IV: 10 mcg/kg
	2–4 years	PO: 35 mcg/kg IV: 35 mcg/kg	PO: 10 mcg/kg IV: 10 mcg/kg
	5–9 years	PO: 25 mcg/kg max dose 750 mcg IV: 25 mcg/kg max dose 500 mcg	PO: 6 mcg/kg max 250 mcg/day IV: 6 mcg/kg max 250 mcg/day
	10–17 years	PO: 0.75–1.5 mg IV: 0.5–1 mg	PO: 62.5–250 mcg IV: 62.5–250 mcg

IV = intravenous; PO = per oral.

Administration	Digoxin is usually administered orally. Intravenous digoxin is used in emergencies and when the oral route in not tolerated. Rapid IV administration should be avoided because there is a risk of **hypertension** and **reduced coronary blood flow**. The solution for infusion is diluted with 0.9% sodium chloride or 5% glucose to a maximum concentration of 62.5 mcg/mL. Loading doses should be given over 30–60 minutes and maintenance dose over 10–20 minutes. When switching from the IV to oral route it may be necessary to increase dose by 20–33% to maintain the same plasma-digoxin concentration.
Side effects and interactions	Common side effects of digoxin include arrhythmias, conduction disturbances, diarrhoea, nausea, vomiting, eosinophilia, rash, dizziness, blurred vision and yellow vision. Prolonged use may cause gynaecomastia.

Digoxin has a **very narrow therapeutic index** and toxicity may occur. In case of toxicity, digoxin should be withdrawn and if serious specialist management is required. The latter involves the **administration of digoxin-specific antibodies**. Hypercalcaemia, hypokalaemia, hypomagnesaemia and hypoxia increase the risk of toxicity. Digoxin is a substrate of P-gp (p-glycoprotein), and inhibitors of P-gp such as **amiodarone** can significantly increase digoxin levels. Digoxin should also be used with caution with drugs that slow AV conduction, such as β-blockers. |
| Monitoring | **Monitoring of drug levels is essential** to avoid digitalis toxicity. Blood should be taken at least 6 hours after a dose. Plasma-digoxin concentration should be kept at 0.8–2 g/L. |
| Cost | Digoxin is **cheap**. The oral solution of digoxin 50 mcg/mL is £5.35 for a 60 mL bottle and a 28-tablet pack of all tablet strengths (62.5 mg, 125 mg and 250 mg) is £1.60. |

Dobutamine

CLINICAL PHARMACOLOGY

Why and when?	Dobutamine is a commonly used **vasopressor sympathomimetic amine** for the management of hypotension. It is a **synthetic catecholamine** developed in 1973 by altering isoprenaline to minimize some of its unwanted adrenergic effects. It stimulates cardiac β_1-adrenergic receptors increasing myocardial contractility and heart rate. It is about four times more potent than dopamine in improving myocardial function and left ventricular output in hypotensive preterm newborns but has less effect on blood pressure. At higher doses its β_2-adrenergic effects lower peripheral vascular resistance. Unlike dopamine, dobutamine is not dependent on the release of endogenous catecholamines for its positive ionotropic effect. Moreover, it does not act on peripheral dopaminergic receptors.
Absorption and distribution	Dobutamine is always administered as intravenous (IV) infusion preferably via a central line although it can be given peripherally, if necessary, for short periods. It does not cross the blood–brain barrier in significant amounts.
Biology	Dobutamine has two main effects a **positive inotropic** and **positive chronotropic** action on heart and a variable peripheral vasodilatory effect mediated via β-adrenergic receptors. It has relatively less affinity for peripheral α-adrenergic receptors as compared with dopamine. Dobutamine leads to more consistent improvement in blood flow and cardiac output. The net desired effect is improved myocardial contractility and left ventricular cardiac output in a hypotensive child. Dobutamine itself has limited α_1 and α_2 activity.

α_1	α_2	β_1	β_2
↑vasoconstriction ↑peripheral vascular resistance	↓insulin release ↓noradrenaline release	↑inotropy ↑chronotropy	↑vasodilation ↑glycogenolysis ↓mediator release

Clearance	Dobutamine clearance is rapid but variable in children. Its plasma **half-life is** usually **5–10 minutes**. Individual assessment is important, and this can be made within 10–15 minutes of starting treatment. Plasma dobutamine is cleared by liver uptake and renal excretion. Care must be exercised when using in children with liver and renal compromise. It is excreted in urine mainly as inactive metabolites.

PRACTICAL PRESCRIBING

Dosing	**Dobutamine is given as an infusion**. Cardiovascular effects are usually seen between 2 and 10 micrograms (mcg)/kg/min. Higher doses (i.e. >20 mcg/kg/min) are usually not tolerated as they lead to tachycardia and reduced ventricular diastole. It is usual practice to start dobutamine infusions at 5 mcg/kg/min and adjust the rate depending on cardiovascular response. If doses over 20 mcg/kg/min are required then a second inotrope can be added or used.
Administration	To give dobutamine it is necessary to make up an infusion. There are many ways of achieving this but in many intensive care units in the UK a 'standard infusion' is used. It is important to check local protocols to reduce the risk of drug errors. One infusion regimen is given below: Add 15 mg/kg body weight and dilute up to 50 mL total volume with 10% glucose or 0.9% saline. Infusing at a rate of 1 mL/h will give an infusion of 5 mcg/kg/min. Dobutamine is inactivated by alkaline solutions and it is incompatible with bicarbonate and alkaline solutions.
Drug errors and safety	**Dobutamine infusion should be preferably used via a central line** but extravasation from peripheral administration does not lead to the tissue damage seen with dopamine. Tachycardia can occur. Pulmonary oedema due to increased pulmonary blood pressure is reported. In general, side effects are uncommon with doses under 15 mcg/kg/min. Drug interactions with β-blockers causing hypertension have been reported. Dobutamine has no known teratogenic effects. Long-term effects are unknown.
Monitoring	Infants requiring dobutamine infusion for hypotension should be on continuous monitoring, including heart rate, blood pressure and regular checks of the site of infusion for blanching or extravasation should be made and documented. High doses can cause tachycardia and arrhythmia. Myocardial function and cardiac output can be monitored using echocardiography.
Cost	Dobutamine **is inexpensive**. A 250 mg/20 mL ampoule costs £5.20.

Docusate

CLINICAL PHARMACOLOGY

Why and when?	The primary indication for docusate in children is **chronic constipation**. It is widely believed to act as a stool softener. It is an important example of a drug that is frequently prescribed but for which there is **little or no good evidence in any age group**. Whilst it is relatively cheap, the frequency of prescription means that it is in fact very costly. In the UK the National Health Service (NHS) spends about £10 million a year (almost £1 million a month) on sodium docusate. It **is probably safe** and in all the studies undertaken has **effects very similar to placebo**. It is recommended for treatment of constipation in children older than 6 months of age who report hard stools. Docusate can also be used as an adjunct for barium meals and in the removal of excess ear wax in adults. There is also little evidence of its effectiveness as a treatment for ear wax removal.
Absorption	Docusate is **not absorbed** and acts locally in the gastrointestinal tract.
Biology	Docusate is **an anionic surfactant** that helps lower the surface tension at the oil–water interface of the stool and thus allows water and lipids or fats to enter the stool. It should not be given at the same time as mineral-oil products like paraffin. The evidence for a significant effect on stool volume or water content in healthy volunteers is lacking, however. It is reported to **work slowly** after oral administration (1–3 days). After rectal administration it works quickly (within 20 minutes), although given the poor evidence for efficacy this may be due to a direct mechanical effect.
Clearance	Docusate is not absorbed to any significant degree and therefore **cleared entirely in the faeces**. The speed of clearance is entirely dependent upon the **gut transit time**, which is typically shorter in early life. The mean gut transit time for UK children under 3 years is about 30 hours and the mean gut transit time for older children is about 36 hours although there is considerable variability between individuals.

PRACTICAL PRESCRIBING

Dosing	Dosing regimens are typically age banded. For children aged **6 months–1 year** the usual prescribed dose is **12.5 mg three times a day**. For children aged **2–11 years** the usual dose is **12.5–25 mg three times a day** using a paediatric oral solution. For older children aged **12–17 years** doses of up to **500 mg a day** can be given in divided doses as either oral solution or capsules.
Administration	Docusate is given usually given orally in children. Rectal preparations are also available. The paediatric oral solution can be mixed with milk, water or squash for administration.
Drug errors and safety	There are **limited side effects** for docusate. It can cause abdominal cramps and nausea. Docusate should be prescribed with caution in combination with stimulant laxatives and liquid paraffin. This can lead to diarrhoea and hypokalaemia.
Monitoring	No monitoring is required.
Cost	Docusate **is relatively cheap**. The oral solution costs around £9 for 300 mL of 10 mg/1 mL solution; it costs around £2 for 30 100 mg capsules. Docusate is also available over the counter. However, it is a significant cost for health economies worldwide.

Domperidone

CLINICAL PHARMACOLOGY

Why and when?	Domperidone is a **prokinetic agent**. It is used to reduce nausea and vomiting by increasing the speed of food moving through the gastrointestinal tract. It is often used in children with **gastroesophageal reflux disease (GORD)** although its use is rooted in historical practice rather than having a strong evidence base. In April 2014, MHRA released advice that domperidone should no longer be prescribed to treat conditions such as gastro-oesophageal reflux and heartburn. **It should now only be used if advised by a specialist**. Domperidone should only be prescribed for the shortest possible duration and only after an ECG is undertaken given the risk of cardiac side effects.
Absorption and distribution	Orally administered, domperidone has a **rapid absorption** with peak levels being reached in c.**1 hour** but a **low bioavailability** (c.15%) due to a **high first-pass metabolism in the gut and liver**. Over 90% of domperidone is bound to plasma proteins and it does not cross the blood–brain barrier.
Biology	Domperidone is a **selective dopamine receptor**-2 and receptor-3 (D_2 and D_3) **antagonist**. Although it does not readily cross the blood–brain barrier it exerts central nervous system effects by acting on the **chemoreceptor trigger zone**, an area in the 4th ventricle that is **outside the blood–brain barrier**. In the gastrointestinal tract, domperidone inhibits D_2 and D_3 receptors in the stomach and duodenum, **increasing peristalsis** and **promoting gastric emptying**. Domperidone also increases constriction of the lower oesophageal sphincter, and thus **reduces reflux** of gastric contents.
Clearance	Domperidone undergoes extensive first-pass metabolism by the cytochrome P450 system in the liver, mainly by **CYP3A4**. Its clearance is significantly altered when used with drugs that either induce or inhibit the CYP3A4 enzymes. **Potent CYP3A4 inhibitors** include **azole antifungals,** e.g. itraconazole and **some macrolides**, e.g. erythromycin and clarithromycin. Moderate inhibitors include diltiazem and verapamil. Some of these drugs also prolong the QT-interval and care must be taken to avoid using other medicines with domperidone. The **half-life in healthy adults is 7–8 hours**.

Drugs that prolong the QTc interval

There is a long list of drugs that prolong the QTc but most are now only rarely used in paediatric practice. Another prokinetic, **cisapride**, was used widely until 2000 but was withdrawn from the UK due to safety concerns. The more commonly encountered drugs in paediatric practice are 'antis'.

Some antidepressants, e.g. **citalopram** or antipsychotics, e.g. **haloperidol**
Antiarrhythmics, e.g. **amiodarone**, **sotalol**
Antibiotics, e.g. **erythromycin.**

PRACTICAL PRESCRIBING

Dosing	Doses are **weight dependent**. For children up to 35 kg usual starting doses are 250 micrograms/kg 3 times a day but it may be increased up to 400 micrograms/kg 3 times a day if there is a suboptimal therapeutic response. For children over 35 kg the dose is 10 mg 3 times a day (maximum dose of 30 mg/day).
Administration	Domperidone is given **orally** in children. This can be via a tablet or oral suspension (1 mg/mL). Although absorption is improved by co-administration with food, **it is usually given before meals** as it promotes gastric emptying.
Drug errors, safety and side effects	Domperidone **prolongs the QT interval** and therefore should be prescribed with caution as this can result **in cardiac arrhythmias** (ventricular tachycardia, fibrillation or torsades de pointes). These effects are particularly prominent with higher doses (>30 mg/day) of domperidone. Domperidone should **not be prescribed** to those with **underlying cardiac disease**, concomitantly with other **QT interval prolonging drugs** or **strong CYP3A4 inhibitors**. Domperidone should also be avoided in those with severe hepatic impairment, and doses should be reduced in mild or moderate hepatic impairment. Dose intervals need to be extended in children with renal impairment. Domperidone also **stimulates prolactin secretion** and can result in galactorrhoea and amenorrhoea.
Monitoring	No formal monitoring of domperidone is required. However, **prior to prescribing an ECG should be performed**. Dosage should be monitored and the lowest possible dose providing symptom relief should be prescribed. It should only be prescribed for a short interval of no longer than 1 week.
Cost	Domperidone in tablet form is **cheap**. 10 mg tablets cost 2–3p each. Oral suspension is more expensive costing around £1 for 10 mL (10 mg).

Calculating the QTc

At higher heart rates it is necessary to use a correction factor to decide if there is a prolonged QT-interval. The most common equation used for QT-interval correction is Bazett's formula, which is:

QTc = QT interval in seconds / duration of the R-R interval in seconds

Whilst long QT syndrome is uncommon it is not rare and affects about 1 in every 2000 children. A QTc of >440 ms for males or >460 ms for females is considered prolonged.

Dopamine

CLINICAL PHARMACOLOGY

Why and when?	Dopamine is a **vasopressor sympathomimetic amine**. It is a naturally occurring catecholamine and precursor of both noradrenaline and adrenaline. It works by stimulating cardiovascular α- and β-adrenergic receptors **as well as dopaminergic receptors** in a dose-dependent way. Stimulation of **α-receptor** leads to vasoconstriction, increase in systemic and pulmonary vascular resistance and blood pressure. **β-receptor** stimulation results in **increased cardiac contractility and rate**. Its overall effects are also influenced by adrenal function, adrenergic receptor expression, myocardial maturity and other local vasodilators, including nitric oxide and prostaglandins.
Absorption and distribution	Dopamine has a short half-life of 5–10 minutes and is always administered as IV infusion through a central line. When given as an IV infusion **dopamine does not cross the blood–brain barrier**.
Biology	Peripheral dopamine is a **potent vasopressor**. It has three main effects: positive inotropic and positive chronotropic action on heart (β_1) and vasoconstriction (α). Lower doses (2–10 microgram (mcg)/kg/min) also improve renal blood flow by dopaminergic receptor (DA_1) stimulation. Its net effect is to increase blood pressure with little or no improvement in systemic or cerebral blood flow.
	Dopamine **increases cardiac output** in doses under 10 mcg/kg/min by stimulating myocardial β_1-receptors. Heart rate increases, and cardiac systole is shorter. Higher doses can lead to more α receptor than β-receptor stimulation. The net effect may be increase in blood pressure due to peripheral vasoconstriction but without further increase in cardiac output and systemic blood flow. In fact the cardiac output may reduce due to myocardial inefficiency and increased afterload. The effects of adrenoreceptor/peripheral dopaminergic receptor activation are listed below:

α_1	α_2	β_1	β_2	DA_1
↑vasoconstriction ↑peripheral vascular resistance	↓insulin release ↓noradrenaline release	↑inotropy ↑chronotropy	↑vasodilation ↑glycogenolysis ↓mediator release	Vasodilation of mesenteric and renal vasculature

Clearance	Up to 50% of infused dopamine is converted to noradrenaline, which can explain more peripheral vasoconstriction due to α_1-receptor stimulation at higher doses. Plasma dopamine is also cleared by liver uptake and renal excretion. Care must be taken when using in children with liver and renal compromise. Its plasma **half-life is 5–10 minutes**. It is excreted in urine mainly as inactive metabolites.

PRACTICAL PRESCRIBING

Dosing	**Dopamine is given as an infusion**. Cardiovascular effects can be seen between 2 and 10 mcg/kg/min dose. Doses above 20 mcg/kg/min can result in severe vasoconstriction and resulting poor tissue perfusion despite improved blood pressure. It is advisable to start at lower doses and assess cardiovascular response in order to titrate the dose.
	It is usually better to add a second inotrope rather than increasing the dose over 20 mcg/kg/min. Tachyphylaxis is well described with dopamine, hence the dose may need increasing over time.
Administration	To give dopamine it is necessary to **make up an infusion**. There are many ways of achieving this but in many intensive care units in the UK a 'standard infusion' is used. It is important to check local protocols to reduce the risk of drug errors. One infusion regime is given below:
	Add 15 mg/kg body weight and dilute up to 50 mL total volume with 10% glucose or 0.9% saline. Infusing at a rate of 1 mL/h will give an infusion of 5 mcg/kg/min.
	Dopamine is inactivated by alkaline solutions and it is incompatible with bicarbonate and alkaline solutions.
Drug errors and safety	**Dopamine infusion should be used with extreme care via a central line** due to extravasation risk when using peripheral veins. If extravasation occurs, stop infusion; gently aspirate extravasated solution (do NOT flush the line); remove needle/cannula; elevate extremity. Initiate phentolamine and apply dry warm compresses.
	Drug interactions with tolazoline and phenytoin causing hypotension have been reported. Dopamine can lead to **suppression of serum TSH, T$_4$** and prolactin levels in very low birth weight neonates.
Monitoring	Infants requiring dopamine infusion for hypotension should be on continuous **heart rate and blood pressure monitoring**. Higher doses can cause tachycardia and arrhythmia. Myocardial function and cardiac output can be monitored using echocardiography.
Cost	**Dopamine is cheap**. A 200 mg (5 mL) ampoule costs around £3.90.

Dornase alfa (DNAse)

CLINICAL PHARMACOLOGY

Why and when?	Dornase alfa is a **nebulized mucolytic** used to aid airway clearance in individuals with cystic fibrosis (CF). It has been shown to **improve lung function and reduce pulmonary exacerbations**. Most guidelines suggest performing airway clearance 30 minutes after the dornase alfa is administered. Dornase alfa is not useful in non-CF bronchiectasis.
Absorption and distribution	Dornase alfa is **only administered via nebulizer** and acts locally on the respiratory tract. Animal studies have demonstrated **minimal systemic absorption**.
Biology	**Dornase alfa is a recombinant human enzyme**, deoxyribonuclease (DNAse), which catalyzes the cleavage of the phosphodiesterase DNA backbone, leading to the **degradation of DNA**. Viscous secretions in the respiratory tract of patients with CF contain high concentrations of extracellular DNA. Dornase alfa cleaves this extracellular DNA, **reducing the viscosity of secretions** and aiding airway clearance.
Clearance	Dornase alfa has an elimination **half-life of 3–4 hours**. The sputum enzyme level peaks 15 minutes post nebulization. The level falls quickly and is <50% of the peak concentration by 2 hours. Despite this, the effects on sputum rheology persist beyond 12 hours.

Nebulizers as a form of drug delivery

Nebulizers are a commonly used method of delivering inhaled medications. To be effective, the drug must be dispersible into a liquid medium. This can then be made into aerosol droplets, which can be inhaled. The particle size significantly influences drug deposition with large particles (>10 microM) landing in the upper airway, medium-sized particles (2–4 microM) landing in the bronchi and bronchioles, and smaller particles depositing in the alveoli. Aerosolization requires a dispersing force (either a jet of gas or ultrasonic waves). All current nebulizers are either (i) jet (or pneumatic) small-volume nebulizers or (ii) ultrasonic or electronic nebulizers. Jet nebulizers use a stream of pressurized gas, whereas ultrasonic and electronic nebulizers use high-frequency acoustic energy and vibrating mesh technology. Electronic nebulizers can be useful in reducing the speed of drug delivery. In many situations it is more efficient to deliver inhaled drugs using a valved holding chamber (spacer device). However, these are not suitable for some inhaled medications and it is difficult to provide additional oxygen to children using spacers. Therefore, nebulizers are still commonly encountered in clinical practice.

PRACTICAL PRESCRIBING

Dosing	For child 5–17 years: 2500 units (2.5 mg) once daily by nebulizer. **Ultrasonic nebulizers are unsuitable for delivery of dornase alfa**.
Administration	Dornase alfa **should be given approximately 30 minutes before chest physiotherapy**. This is often difficult for children and families to build into a daily routine and significantly impacts on adherence. It is supplied in 2.5 mL vials and should be used undiluted.
Side effects and interactions	Side effects from dornase alfa are **rare** but include chest pain, dyspnoea, dyspepsia, dysphonia, conjunctivitis, fever, skin reactions and increased risk of infection.
Monitoring	**No monitoring required**. Benefits are usually seen within 2 weeks of initiating treatment, but a longer trial of treatment may be indicated in severe disease.
Cost	In keeping with many medicines useful for CF, dornase alfa is expensive. 1 months' supply costs approximately £500. Additional costs include the need for a nebulizer device. These vary in design and efficiency but newer devices, such as electronic nebulizers which are quicker to use, can be very expensive and equipment costs are often not met by the NHS in the UK.

Erythromycin

CLINICAL PHARMACOLOGY

Why and when?	Erythromycin is a macrolide antibiotic. It has a broad spectrum of activity. Macrolides have a similar but not identical antibacterial spectrum to penicillin and are an alternative in **penicillin-allergic patients**. It is particularly used when treating **atypical lower respiratory tract infections**. Erythromycin is used for *Campylobacter* enteritis, respiratory infections (pneumonia, whooping cough, *Legionella*, *Chlamydia* and *Mycoplasma* infection) and skin infections. It has poor activity against *Haemophilus influenzae*. Erythromycin increases gastrointestinal motility and may decrease gastric emptying time in some individuals, which can be of therapeutic value.
Absorption and distribution	Oral erythromycin has a **relatively fast speed of absorption** (peak serum concentration within 1 hour) but poor oral bioavailability of 30–40%. The bioavailability is reduced by gastric acid and hence it is administered as enteric-coated or esterified form. After absorption, **erythromycin diffuses readily** into most bodily fluids and is 75–95% protein bound. In the absence of meningeal inflammation it does not readily cross the blood-brain barrier.
Biology	Erythromycin is a **protein synthesis inhibitor** and binds 50S ribosomal subunits of susceptible organisms. Its binding inhibits peptidyl transferase activity and interferes with translocation of amino acids during translation and assembly of proteins. It can be **bacteriostatic or bactericidal** depending on the organism and drug concentration.
Clearance	Erythromycin is concentrated in the liver and excreted in bile. It is extensively metabolized and after oral administration less than 5% of the administered dose can be found in the active form in urine. The **half-life is short** ranging **between 0.8 and 3 hours**.
Dosing	The dose of erythromycin and frequency of administration are dependent on the age of the child, severity and source of infection. It is usually given **four times a day** and ideally should be given on an **empty stomach**, with each dose at least 3 hours apart. Typical doses are 125 mg 6-hourly for children aged 1–23 months, 250 mg 6-hourly for children aged 2–7 years and 500 mg 6-hourly for older children although doses are usually doubled in severe infection. A reduced dose is recommended in severe renal impairment due to risk of ototoxicity. Lower doses are given when it is used as a prokinetic agent or as antibiotic prophylaxis.

PRACTICAL PRESCRIBING

Administration	Erythromycin is most commonly given orally and is available as capsules (250 mg), tablets (250 and 500 mg) or as a sugar-free liquid suspension (125 mg/5 mL, 250 mg/5 mL and 500 mg/5 mL). Occasionally erythromycin is given intravenously. In this case the reconstituted solution needs to be diluted in glucose 5% (neutralized with sodium bicarbonate) or sodium chloride 0.9% to a concentration of 1–5 mg/mL and to be given over 20–60 minutes. **Higher concentrations up to 10 mg/mL can be given but only via a central venous catheter**.
Side effects and contraindications	In babies under 2 weeks of age, it increases the risk of hypertrophic **pyloric stenosis**. The mechanism of action is unknown but it increases the risk of pyloric stenosis significantly (8- to 30-fold), possibly through an interaction with gastric motilin receptors. It is best avoided in late pregnancy and in the early postpartum period as erythromycin crosses the placenta and enters breast milk in small amounts. Fetal drug levels reach 5–20% of maternal serum concentrations and are associated with a non-significant increase in the risk of pyloric stenosis when taken during the last trimester. Gastrointestinal side effects are common, especially **nausea, vomiting** and **diarrhoea**. These occur most frequently at higher doses.
	Rarely, macrolide antibiotics can cause cholestatic jaundice, hepatotoxicity, rash, colitis, arrhythmias, pancreatitis, QT-prolongation, Stevens–Johnson syndrome and toxic epidermal necrolysis. In large doses reversible hearing loss and tinnitus may occur but the frequency of this is unknown.
Interactions and monitoring	Erythromycin is metabolized by the **CYP3A family**. Drugs which may induce or inhibit this enzyme family can impair the clinical impact of erythromycin and cause increased risk of side effects associated with either erythromycin or the interacting drug. Commonly encountered drugs with known or theoretical interactions include carbamazepine, digoxin, furosemide and midazolam. Steroids, aminophylline and bronchodilators all interact with erythromycin to result in increased **hypokalaemia** and so it should be used with **care in acute asthma**. It should be avoided when using with other drugs that **prolong the QT interval,** e.g. domperidone, flecainide and ondansetron.
Cost	Erythromycin is fairly **cheap** and cheaper than some of the newer macrolides like azithromycin. The cost is dependent on formulation; it can be as low as £1.25 for 28 250 mg tablets. Oral suspension is around £5–6 for 100 mL of 125 mg/5 mL or 250 mg/5 mL. Intravenous preparations are considerably more expensive (£18–23 per 1 g ampoule).

79

Ethosuximide

CLINICAL PHARMACOLOGY

Why and when?	Ethosuximide is **an antiepileptic drug** (AED) and a member of the succinimide family. It differs from other AEDs in that it **blocks a particular type of calcium channel** that is active in **primary generalized epilepsies**. It is often the first-line medication for **childhood absence epilepsy** but has no effect against (or **may even worsen**) partial and tonic-clonic seizures. For this reason, its main use is among younger children where this type of epilepsy predominates.

Some older children who have absence seizures have more complicated disorders that are harder to treat and may not be outgrown, such as atypical absence or juvenile myoclonic epilepsy. These children may also have other types of seizures and have a different electroencephalogram (EEG) pattern than children with typical childhood absence epilepsy. Ethosuximide can be effective in controlling absence seizures in many of these children, but other medications often are needed to control other types of seizures. It can also be useful as an **adjunctive medication** for patients with **juvenile myoclonic epilepsy and Lennox–Gastaut syndrome**.

Absorption	Ethosuximide is well absorbed from the gut, with **bioavailability** following oral administration of **>90%**. It is not bound to plasma proteins. Peak plasma levels are reached in 3–5 hours after administration of a tablet; this may be shorter when syrup is used.
Biology	The exact mechanism of action of ethosuximide is **not entirely understood**, but it does not appear to alter brain **γ-aminobutyric acid** (GABA) concentrations. Ethosuximide inhibits NADPH-linked aldehyde reductase necessary for the formation of γ-hydroxybutyrate (a precursor of GABA), which has been associated with the induction of absence seizures.

It also inhibits the Na^+-K^+ ATPase system and has been shown to decrease non-inactivating Na^+ currents in thalamocortical neurons, as well as **blocking Ca^{2+}-dependent K^+ channels.** This leads to a decrease of the burst firing of thalamocortical neurons and may explain the anti-absence seizure activity of the drug.

Clearance	Ethosuximide undergoes extensive metabolism in the liver and the **half-life is long**, about **30–40 hours in children and 50–60 hours in adults**. In children, steady state is reached after 6 days of taking a stable dose.

There are no studies on the effect of renal insufficiency on the pharmacokinetics of ethosuximide. Renal insufficiency is unlikely to greatly alter clearance because about 80% is cleared via the liver and only 20% via the kidney. Those with liver disease may need to be started at a lower dose and have their dosage increased more slowly.

PRACTICAL PRESCRIBING

Dosing	For **oral** administration, it is introduced at a dose of **5 mg/kg twice daily** (max per dose 125 mg) for children aged from 1 month to 5 years. The dose is gradually increased every 5–7 days with the **maintenance dose usually between 20 mg and 40 mg/kg/day** in two divided doses. In older children (6–17 years) the dose is initially **250 mg twice daily**, increased in steps of 250 mg every 5–7 days with the **usual maintenance dose of 500–750 mg twice daily**, up to 1 g twice daily if needed.
	The optimal daily dose of 20 mg/kg gives average plasma levels within the accepted therapeutic range of 40–100 mcg/mL. Levels are not usually monitored **unless non-compliance is suspected**, as seizure response is best used as a guide to treatment success.
Side effects and considerations	Ethosuximide is **usually well tolerated** in children, with the most common side effects being gastrointestinal. These include nausea, abdominal discomfort, vomiting, anorexia and diarrhoea. Most often these **can be helped by dividing the daily dosage into smaller doses** to be **taken with meals.**
	Less commonly children may seem less alert than normal, and may say they cannot think clearly, or their coordination may be affected. They may also have changes in mood or become irritable more easily. Some children taking ethosuximide develop **persistent headaches**, which do not appear to be dose related. There is also a very small risk of blood abnormalities, so patients/parents should be warned to look for sore throat, fever, sores in the mouth or easy bruising.
	The most common idiosyncratic reaction to ethosuximide is a mild rash, which often disappears if the medication is stopped. As with many seizure medicines, skin rashes (including the very rare Stevens–Johnson syndrome, which can be fatal) have been a problem for a small number of patients.
	The level of ethosuximide is reduced if it is taken concurrently with enzyme-inducing medications, some of these include carbamazepine, phenytoin, phenobarbital and rifampin. Specific advice is available for its use in pregnancy weighing up risk and benefit. It is secreted in breastmilk and estimates are that a nursing infant might receive a dose of 13–38 mg per day. The effect of this dose on an infant is unknown.
	Treatment should not be discontinued abruptly as seizures may be precipitated. It should be tapered over a period of 5–6 weeks. Patient information for parents is available at https://www.medicinesforchildren.org.uk/ethosuximide-preventing-seizures.
Cost	Ethosuximide is available as both an oral suspension and capsules. The treatment cost is **moderately expensive** with the oral suspension costing £173 per 200 mL.

Fluticasone

CLINICAL PHARMACOLOGY

Why and when?	Fluticasone propionate is best known for its use in the **prophylaxis for asthma** and is introduced on the second and third step on the *ladder* of asthma management. It is used to **prevent** asthma exacerbations and not used for management of acute asthma. Fluticasone is also used topically in the prophylaxis and treatment of rhinitis, in nasal polyps and inflammatory skin conditions.
Absorption	Inhaled fluticasone is absorbed via the lungs into the systemic circulation. The typical systemic bioavailability of inhaled fluticasone propionate after inhalation is 20–30% in healthy subjects but lower in children with asthma (c.5–10%). Fluticasone is metabolized by CYP3A5 in the lung. The remainder of the inhaler dose, approximately 80%, is swallowed. Fluticasone is then metabolized by CYP3A4, which lines the gastrointestinal tract; therefore, the majority of fluticasone goes through **extensive first-pass metabolism** and, theoretically, very little is absorbed to the systemic circulation. Fluticasone applied topically has a variable absorption due to many factors including skin integrity. Intranasal bioavailability is less than 2%, and as discussed above, oral bioavailability is minimal due its extensive metabolism in the gastrointestinal tract. Fluticasone that does get absorbed into the systemic circulation is metabolized in the liver by CYP3A4; this is its main circulating metabolite.
Biology	Fluticasone is a **potent synthetic corticosteroid**, which is a vasoconstrictor and an anti-inflammatory. It binds to intracellular glucocorticoid receptors. Fluticasone's exact mechanism of action is not fully understood but its binding to the glucocorticoid receptor leads to **altered protein synthesis**, reduced capillary permeability, kinin and histamine release. The **glucocorticoid receptor complex** downregulates proinflammatory mediators (interleukin-1, -3, -5) and upregulates anti-inflammatory mediators (IκB). These effects help symptoms and contribute to a reduction in asthma attacks. When used in treatment-naïve children, symptoms will resolve at different rates and patients should be warned to **expect improvement slowly** (over weeks rather than days).
Clearance	Clearance depends upon route of administration. When inhaled, much of the dose will be swallowed and excreted unchanged in the faeces. Fluticasone that reaches the lungs will be absorbed over 2–3 hours and make its way into the blood where it is highly protein bound (>90%). Once in the circulation is mostly cleared in the liver. Fluticasone propionate has extensive distribution into tissues; with a high volume of distribution, it has a relatively long **half-life** of between **8 and 12 hours**.

PRACTICAL PRESCRIBING

Dosing	For use in asthma the dose varies between 50 and 250 mcg/puff. It is usually given as **one or two puffs twice a day**. The usual starting dose in a child is 50–100 mcg twice a day, and the maximum licensed dose in children under 16 years old is 200 mcg twice a day. Higher doses may be prescribed to those over 16 years of age. Children <12 years taking **more than 200 mcg** of fluticasone per day are in **high dose range**.
Administration	For use in childhood respiratory disease it is administered via an inhaler. This can either be via a pressurized metered dose inhaler (pMDI) with a spacer (such as Flixotide Evohaler), as a dry powder inhaler (DPI) (Flixotide Accuhaler) or as a combination inhaler with long-acting β_2-agonist salmeterol (Seretide Accuhaler or Evohaler). Administration for use in nasal polyps is by intranasal drops, and for use in skin conditions it is applied topically as a cream.
Drug errors and safety	Care should be taken when changing from beclomethasone to fluticasone as there is a **doubling in strength for a given dose**. The dose needs to be regularly reviewed and be given at the lowest possible therapeutic dose. Common side effects are oral thrush, sore throat and tongue, and hoarseness. It is advised to wash the mouth out with water after administration of the drug via an inhaler (or **brush your teeth**). Generic corticosteroid side effects also still occur including difficulty sleeping, excitability and irritability, anxiety, depression, arthralgia, indigestion, hyperglycaemia, and cataracts. In those taking high doses this can lead to **adrenal suppression**, which can present as acute adrenal crisis. A *steroid card* should therefore be carried by all those on high dose steroids. Long-term corticosteroid use is also known to lead to reduction in bone mineral density. **Growth restriction** is a known side effect and of particular consideration in the paediatric population, although this is usually only transient as disease-related growth restriction is removed.
Monitoring	In patients on long-term corticosteroid treatment it is important to monitor for side effects. **Growth should be monitored** and adrenal suppression should be screened for in those with poor growth on high steroid doses (or dual sources of steroids, e.g. nasal steroids as well). In asthma patients when they are reviewed, ensure that they are using their **inhalation device correctly**, using it at the right dose and at the correct times of day. Adherence and ability to use the device should be monitored before considering increasing the dose of the inhaler. Always recommend the use of a spacer device to improve drug delivery in children using pMDIs.
Cost	Fluticasone is **relatively expensive** with inhaled preparations varying from c.£4 to almost £60 depending on the dose and strength. It is more costly than beclometasone propionate preparations. The cost of pMDIs is usually cheaper per dose than equivalent DPIs but there are some exceptions. pMDIs should only be used with an appropriate spacer device (**valved holding chamber**).

83

Furosemide

CLINICAL PHARMACOLOGY

Why and when?	Furosemide is a **loop diuretic** that is used to treat **volume overload** in congestive heart failure, renal disease, hepatic disease, pulmonary oedema and often following cardiac surgery. It does this by increasing the amount of urine that is produced by the kidneys and lowering the amount of circulating volume in the body. Furosemide can be used alone or with other medications to manage **hypertension** in children. It is also sometimes used long term in neonates with **chronic lung disease**.
Absorption and distribution	Furosemide is usually **rapidly absorbed** from the gastrointestinal tract; however, only 60–70% is absorbed and this is mainly in the upper duodenum. Once absorbed it is largely (c.95%) **bound to albumin** where the peak effects occur within **1–2 hours** and duration of action is roughly 4 hours. Absorption of oral furosemide can be impaired in children with significant oedema. It is believed that oedematous duodenum is less efficient at absorbing furosemide and children who are unresponsive to oral dosing **may require intravenous treatment** until fluid balance is restored.
Biology	Loop diuretics earn their name by acting directly in the **loop of Henle** in renal tubules. Furosemide inhibits the reabsorption of fluid from the thick ascending limb of the loop of Henle, by affecting the transport of sodium, potassium and chloride. It works directly on the **$Na^+/K^+/2Cl^-$ co-transporter** and causes a halt in the transport of these electrolytes across the renal tubules. **Reabsorption of sodium and chloride from the nephron is reduced**, which ultimately **increases** the production **hypotonic or isotonic urine**.
Clearance	Furosemide is mostly eliminated by the kidneys (up to 90%) with a very small proportion cleared by the hepatobiliary system (10–15%). It has a **half-life of 1.5–2.0 hours** in most children and adults but may be variable and significantly longer (even >24 hours) in preterm infants of low gestational age.
Dosing	The dose and frequency of administration is dependent on the age of the child, weight of the child, severity of fluid overload, renal function and route of administration. A typical recommended oral dose is **0.5–2 mg/kg** repeated every 12–24 hours in neonates and every 8–12 hours in older children and adults. In children aged 1 month to 11 years, the maximum recommended oral dose is 12 mg/kg/day or 80 mg/day (whichever is lower). Children older than this can take up to 120 mg/day. If given intravenously, the recommended dose is usually 0.5–1 mg/kg. The maximum recommended dose is 6 mg/kg in children less than 11 years. Higher doses (more than 50 mg) should be given as an infusion and the maximum recommended daily dose in older children and adults is 1.5 g.

PRACTICAL PRESCRIBING

Administration	For oral use, furosemide can be taken as **tablets** or as an **oral solution**. Tablets can be taken whole or crushed and dissolved in water. In some cases injection solutions can be given by mouth.
	Intravenous injections should be given **over 5–10 minutes**. Slower IV injections can be given in renal impairment. For IV infusions, dilute with 0.9% normal saline to a concentration of 1–2 mg furosemide per 1 mL of 0.9% saline.
Side effects and interactions	Adverse effects of furosemide include **depletion of total body sodium** causing hyponatraemia or extracellular volume depletion. This can lead to hypotension, reduced eGFR and acute kidney injury. **Hypokalaemia** can also occur with prolonged loop diuretic use. This is particularly dangerous in children with hepatic failure as this can precipitate hepatic encephalopathy. In children with low potassium, supplements or concomitant use of potassium-sparing diuretics like amiloride should be considered. Furosemide can also cause **urinary retention** in children with urinary outflow obstruction. Care must be taken to only initiate furosemide treatment if there is established urinary output. There is a risk of **ototoxicity** in children on high doses. This can be reduced by dividing administration of higher doses. Non-steroidal anti-inflammatory drugs (NSAIDs) should be avoided or used with caution in children on loop diuretics as these will attenuate the effects of furosemide and diuretics may enhance the nephrotoxicity of NSAIDs. **Nephrocalcinosis** is common, particularly in neonates and babies with long-term use. Uncommonly furosemide will cause thrombocytopenia and rarely eosinophilia, leukopenia or bone marrow suppression.
Monitoring	Serum electrolytes, including **sodium**, **potassium**, **chloride** and **creatinine**, should be monitored. In long-term use also consider monitoring of magnesium, calcium, bicarbonate and uric acid, particularly in children with hepatic impairment. Furosemide is ototoxic, particularly when high doses are given rapidly to neonates and hearing tests should be considered. Neonates receiving long courses of furosemide should have **renal ultrasound scans** to check for nephrocalcinosis.
Cost	Furosemide is fairly cheap. Oral furosemide is available in 20 mg tablets, 40 mg tablets and oral solution. Tablets are usually cheaper. A pack of 28 20 mg tablets costs between £0.37 and £1.02. As with other medicines, the differing available concentrations of oral solutions are a potential cause of significant harm. **Great care needs to be taken to ensure that the correct strength is both prescribed and dispensed to parents**. Oral solution furosemide is available in concentrations of 20 mg/5 mL, 40 mg/5 mL and 50 mg/5 mL. A 150 mL bottle furosemide costs between £12 and £20 depending on strength and brand. Intravenous furosemide is very cheap and is available in 10 mg/mL ampoules. A pack of 10 ampoules roughly costs £0.25.

Gabapentin

CLINICAL PHARMACOLOGY

Why and when?	Gabapentin is used in the **treatment of epilepsy**. It is a newer antiepileptic drug (AED), having been used in children since the turn of the 21st century. Unlike some AEDs, it is helpful in only a fairly narrow range of seizure types. It is mainly used to treat **focal seizures**, with or without secondary generalization as either monotherapy or as an adjunct to other AEDs. It has to be used with care as it can worsen absence and myoclonic seizures.
	It is now also used for the **treatment of neuropathic pain in children**. It has also been used for **restless legs syndrome** and **anxiety**. It has modest anti-spastic effects.
Absorption	The absorption of gabapentin from the intestine depends on the L-amino acid carrier system and shows the property of *saturability*, which means that **increasing the dose does not proportionately increase the amount absorbed**. This makes gabapentin relatively safe and free of side effects associated with overdosing. Pregabalin, an analogue of gabapentin, has a much higher bioavailability and remains at around 90% irrespective of the dosage.
Biology	The mechanism for the anticonvulsant and analgesic actions of gabapentin is not well understood. Despite its name and structure, which resembles the neurotransmitter γ-aminobutyric acid (GABA), gabapentin has **little or no activity at central GABA$_A$ or GABA$_B$ receptors**. Gabapentin (and pregabalin) inhibits calcium influx and subsequent release of excitatory neurotransmitters, **selectively inhibiting a subset of voltage-gated calcium channels**. These channels are expressed widely in human tissues.
	The analgesic effect of gabapentin appears to result from prevention of both allodynia (the pain response to normally innocuous stimuli) and hyperalgesia (an exaggerated response to painful stimuli).
Clearance	Gabapentin and pregabalin are predominantly **renally excreted**. They are mostly excreted unchanged in the urine. They must be used with care in patients whose renal function is impaired. Despite the similarity in structure to GABA, gabapentin does not appear to be metabolized into GABA. Its plasma half-life is about 6 hours and **it is not metabolized by the liver**. Unlike many other AEDs it does not induce or inhibit hepatic metabolism of other drugs.

PRACTICAL PRESCRIBING

Dosing	When used as an **adjunctive treatment for focal seizures** the usual oral dose is age and weight dependent. It is usual to gradually increase the dose.
	In children 2–11 years the starting dose is 10 mg/kg once daily on day 1, then 10 mg/kg twice daily on day 2, then 10 mg/kg 3 times a day on day 3. The usual target dose is 30-70 mg/kg daily in children 2-5 years and 25-35 mg/kg daily in children 6-11 years split into 3 doses. The dose must be titrated to response. Some will require longer intervals between dose increases, in some weekly increases may be required.
	In those 12 years and over the initial dose is usually 300 mg 3 times a day. This is then increased in steps of 300 mg every 2–3 days (or sometimes weekly intervals) in 3 divided doses, adjusted according to response. The usual treatment dose is 0.9–3.6 g daily in 3 divided doses (max. per dose 1.6 g 3 times a day).
	Whilst not licensed for the treatment of neuropathic pain, it is used for this indication in children and trials are taking place for this indication. Gabapentin is usually started at a low dose given at night and if tolerated, increased to twice a day then three times a day as directed by an experienced clinician.
Administration	Gabapentin is available as oral solution in a concentration of 50 mg/mL. It is also available as 100 mg, 300 mg and 400 mg capsules, along with 600 mg and 800 mg tablets. Antacids should be avoided within 2 hours before or after taking gabapentin, as they reduce absorption.
Side effects and considerations for use	When starting treatment a child may be **drowsy, dizzy** or **unsteady**. It may have an effect on **appetite**, which can be significant. Children may feel less hungry or have nausea and vomit. A child may also be hungrier than usual and this effect can last for many months. It is helpful to discuss this when starting treatment and advise them to eat food that is low in fat and sugar; otherwise they may put on a lot of weight.
	Diarrhoea, constipation, wind, indigestion or a dry mouth may be experienced and other medicines to help with these symptoms can be prescribed if they are a problem. Occasionally children may seem particularly emotional, anxious or overactive or may have problems with their memory. Usually these effects settle in the first few weeks.
Cost	**Tablets of gabapentin are relatively cheap** with 100 tablets costing around £6–14. The cost for 150 mL of the oral 50 mg/mL solution is higher at £68.

Gastrografin®

CLINICAL PHARMACOLOGY

Why and when?	Gastrografin® is a water-soluble solution containing sodium amidotrizoate and meglumine amidotrizoate. It can be used as **contrast medium** for radiological examinations of the gastrointestinal tract or **an osmotic laxative** for the treatment of uncomplicated meconium ileus and **distal intestinal obstruction syndrome** (DIOS).
Absorption and distribution	Gastrografin is **sparingly absorbed** from the intact gastrointestinal tract enabling its use as a contrast medium.
Biology	As with other contrast media, Gastrografin contains **high concentrations of organically bound iodine**. The high atomic weight of iodine imparts sufficient radiodensity to enable contrast with surrounding tissues. The high osmolarity of Gastrografin draws water into the bowel from surrounding tissues by osmosis. This rehydrates and dissolves inspissated meconium/stool.
Clearance	Only a small fraction of Gastrografin is absorbed from the gastrointestinal tract. When this occurs it is **cleared by the kidneys**, which can result in incidental visualization of the urinary tract.
Dosing	Uncomplicated **meconium ileus** is treated with a single 15–30 mL dose of Gastrografin per rectum.
	DIOS is treated with a single 15–100 mL (depending on age/weight) dose of Gastrografin by mouth or rectum. DIOS is treated with a single dose of 15-30 mL for a child 1-23 months, 50 mL for those weighing 15-25 kg and 100 mL for those weighing 26 kg and above.
	When used as a contrast media, the dose of Gastrografin should be decided by the radiologist performing the investigation.

PRACTICAL PRESCRIBING

Administration	Gastrografin can be administered orally or rectally. When administered orally it should be diluted with two (child >25 kg) or three times (child <25 kg) its volume of water or fruit juice. Clinical experience suggests that it is truly horrible to taste. **Even stoic children and young adults find it unpalatable and some will elect to have a nasogastric tube passed rather than endure its taste**. When given by rectum it should be diluted with four (child >5 years) or five (child <5 years) times its volume of water. Rectal administration should occur slowly under radiological supervision.
Side effects and interactions	The osmotic laxative effect of Gastrografin can cause significant fluid loss from the bowel. Patients must be well hydrated and have electrolyte imbalances corrected prior to treatment. In patients with pre-existing hyperthyroidism, the iodine content of Gastrografin absorbed from the gastrointestinal tract can interfere with thyroid function and **induce a thyrotoxic crisis**.
	In neonates, the absorbed iodine can cause **hypothyroidism**. This risk is higher in preterm infants. Systemic hypersensitivity is mostly mild and occurs generally in the form of skin reactions. Hypersensitivity reactions can occur. These are usually limited to skin reactions but severe reactions have been reported.
Monitoring	**In neonates** and those with **hyperthyroidism** it is recommended that **thyroid function is monitored** after Gastrografin is administered.
Cost	100 mL of Gastrografin costs approximately £15.

Gaviscon®

CLINICAL PHARMACOLOGY

Why and when?	Gaviscon® is used for **gastro-oesophageal reflux disease** (GORD). It forms a layer over acidic stomach contents to stop it refluxing up the oesophagus. There are two preparations, Gaviscon and infant Gaviscon. The latter has a **lower sodium content** and is recommended for use in children up to 1 year of age.
	The National Institute for Health and Care Excellence (NICE) guidelines for suspected infantile GORD recommend a **2-week trial** of infant Gaviscon for infants with **frequent regurgitation and marked distress**. Bottle-fed infants should attempt a reduction in feed volume/frequency and use pre-thickened feed before use. If a 2-week trial of infant Gaviscon is effective at reducing symptoms, parents are advised to try stopping Gaviscon at regular intervals (NICE recommends fortnightly). Gaviscon is also frequently used in older children and adults.
Absorption	Gaviscon is **not absorbed** into the systemic circulation.
Biology	The active ingredient is sodium alginate, a linear polymer of sugar-like monomers. It relies on exposure to **acid stomach contents** to be effective. On contact with gastric acid, alginate precipitates into a viscous gel with near neutral pH. Carbon dioxide is released on contact with stomach acid. This gas forms bubbles in the gel which causes it to float on the top of the gastric contents like a raft. This helps acidic gastric acid to remain in the stomach where it is less likely to cause symptoms. Gaviscon is **not an effective antacid** and whilst it raises the stomach pH slightly the effect is negligible. Gaviscon should relieve symptoms within 30 minutes of administration.
Clearance	The duration of action of infant Gaviscon is variable and depends on a number of factors including the speed of gastric emptying. Both preparations of Gaviscon are cleared in the stool.

PRACTICAL PRESCRIBING

Dosing	The dose and preferred preparation depend on **age and weight**. For infants (children <12 months) infant powder sachets are recommended. Infants <4.5 kg should have one dose (half a dual sachet) to be taken with or after feeds up to six times per day. Heavier infants (> 4.5 kg) should have two doses (2 × half a dual sachet). These heavier infants can have up to 12 doses per day. For older children using Gaviscon liquid, the usual dose is 2.5–5 mL after meals and at bedtime for children of 1–5 years, and 5–10 mL to be taken after meals and at bedtime for children of 6–11 years. Older children and young adults should have 10–20 mL after meals and at bedtime. Gaviscon tablets are available and one tablet contains the equivalent of 5 mL of Gaviscon liquid.
Administration	For breastfed babies, mix the powder with 5 mL of cool boiled water to make a paste; then mix this with a further 10 mL of water. Administer after a breast feed using a syringe or spoon. For bottle-fed babies, add the powder into the feed in the bottle and shake well. For babies weighing up to 4.5 kg (10 lb) mix into at least 115 mL (roughly 4oz) of formula and for babies more than 4.5 kg (10 mL), mix into at least 225 mL (roughly 7.5 oz) of formula.
Contraindications	Gaviscon should be avoided or omitted in individuals with **diarrhoea** or other conditions where **excessive water loss** is likely. It should also be avoided in suspected (or confirmed) intestinal obstruction. Gaviscon contains sodium and this should be taken into account in children with renal impairment, or others on a low-sodium diet.
Drug errors, safety and side effects	Gaviscon frequently causes **constipation** and parents should be made aware of this risk prior to commencing therapy. In other respects Gaviscon is generally well tolerated and very safe. If overdose occurs there is a theoretical possibility of hypomagnesaemia but toxicity is widely regarded to be very low. Care should be taken to avoid medication errors. It should be explained to parents that one dose equals half a dual sachet, not both sides.
Monitoring	Dose can be titrated to response and the **minimum effective dose should be used**. In babies, who will naturally outgrow reflux, the treatment should be periodically stopped to ascertain if it is still necessary.
Cost	Whilst Gaviscon is relatively cheap, its effectiveness is limited and regurgitation is ubiquitous in babies. **Infant Gaviscon is more expensive.** NICE estimates that 30 days' treatment costs c.£22. As more than 250,000 infants will experience reflux symptoms annually in England, prescribing should be limited to those with more severe symptoms or complications. Gaviscon can be bought over the counter for roughly £4 for 24 tablets, or £4 for a 300 mL bottle. Gaviscon infant can also be bought over the counter.

Gentamicin

CLINICAL PHARMACOLOGY

Why and when?

Gentamicin is an **aminoglycoside antibiotic** commonly used for the treatment of infections and surgical prophylaxis. Aminoglycosides are most effective against **aerobic bacteria**. They work **synergistically with β-lactam antibiotics** and are often used in combination with them. Penicillin will provide cover against streptococci. Anaerobic cover can be enhanced with metronidazole. Gentamicin is commonly used in combination with other antibiotics to treat **pyelonephritis/ complex urinary tract infection, severe sepsis, biliary and intra-abdominal infections** and **endocarditis**. It can be nebulized for children with chronic lung infections. Gentamicin can also be 'locked' into a central line to treat lumen infections. Drops are available for bacterial eye, skin and external ear infections.

Absorption

Gentamicin is very **poorly absorbed from the gut**. In treating infections it is usually given by injection (IV or IM). It may be used topically for skin or ear/eye infections. The lack of absorption can be helpful and oral gentamicin can be used to treat **bacterial overgrowth of the gut**. Following IV administration **peak concentrations are reached quickly** (30–60 min). Aminoglycosides are not distributed into adipose tissue, as they are **highly hydrophilic**. Gentamicin has **very poor central nervous system (CNS) penetration** and does not readily cross the blood–brain barrier. Historically, it was used with ampicillin to treat *Listeria* meningitis in neonates but its effectiveness for this is unclear.

Biology

Aminoglycosides act **by inhibiting protein synthesis**. Once inside the bacterial cell, they **bind to the 30S subunit of the ribosome** causing misreading of mRNA, resulting in interruption of normal bacterial protein synthesis. Aminoglycoside uptake into bacteria is via an **oxygen-dependent transport system**. Streptococci and anaerobic bacteria do not have this system. β-lactam antibiotics (active against cell wall) facilitate aminoglycoside cellular penetration, increasing efficacy. Gentamicin is **bactericidal**. Gentamicin exerts **rapid concentration-dependent killing** of sensitive bacteria and has a significant post-antibiotic effect. Single daily dosing appears to be safe, efficacious and cost-effective, and is used in older children.

Clearance

Gentamicin is excreted, unmodified, by the kidneys. It follows classic first-order kinetics and has a usual **plasma half-life of 2–3 hours** in older children and adults. The half-life, however, is **quite variable**, even in individuals with normal renal function. In individuals with impaired renal function, the half-life may be considerably longer. **It is longer in neonates and younger children**.

In obese or severely oedematous patients, use ideal weight for height to calculate the dose: http://www.calculator.net/ideal-weight-calculator.html

PRACTICAL PRESCRIBING

Dosing	**Neonates**: <7 days with normal renal function: **5 mg/kg every 36 hours** by slow IV infusion over 30 min. >7 days to 28 days with normal renal function: **5 mg/kg once daily** by slow IV infusion over 30 min. **Over 1 month**: Initially **7 mg/kg (max. 480 mg) IV once daily** by infusion over at least 30 min. <u>Then adjust according to serum gentamicin concentration</u>. If there is renal impairment the inter-interval period must be increased and in severe renal failure the dose should be decreased; specialist advice is required. Nebulized gentamicin is occasionally used in cystic fibrosis (CF) for chronic *Pseudomonas* or staphylococcal infection but has been mostly supplanted by newer aminoglycosides (tobramycin).
Administration	Gentamicin can be given as an IV infusion, IM injection or rarely, intraventricularly/intrathecally. It can also be used topically in eye or ear infection and as an inhalation. For IV infusion, dilute in 5% glucose or 0.9% sodium chloride solution and give over 30 min. For intrathecal (IT) injection, use preservative-free IT preparations only. For nebulization, dilute preservative-free preparation in 3 mL sodium chloride 0.9%. Administer after physiotherapy. Because of the different regimens there is a **high risk for medication errors to occur**. Many units have specific charts or stickers for prescribing of gentamicin locally. Care should be taken when prescribing and **local guidance always consulted.**
Side effects and interactions	Gentamicin can commonly cause serious dose-related side effects including **nephrotoxicity** and **irreversible hearing loss**. Other uncommon side effects are skin reactions, nausea and vomiting, antibiotic-associated colitis, blood disorders, mood disturbance, liver toxicity, neurotoxicity and stomatitis. Care must be taken in children with muscular weakness as aminoglycosides may **impair neuromuscular transmission**. Dehydration should be corrected before starting gentamicin whenever possible, and parenteral treatment should not exceed 7 days.
Monitoring	Serum concentration of gentamicin **must be measured** in children receiving parenteral gentamicin. In once-daily regimens **trough levels** should be taken at 18–24 hours after the first or second dose (depending on clinical situation) and should be <1 mg/L. If the pre-dose concentration is high, the interval between doses must be increased and renal function should be checked.
Cost	Gentamicin is **inexpensive**. IT preparations are slightly more expensive at c.£1.50/mg (as 5 mg/1 mL ampoules). Gentamicin eye/ear drops solution (0.3%) costs £2.63 for 10 mL. An 80 mg/mL prepared infusion bag costs around £4. Higher concentrations cost a similar amount per mg of gentamicin.

Glycopyrronium bromide (glycopyrrolate)

CLINICAL PHARMACOLOGY

Why and when?	Glycopyrronium bromide is an **anticholinergic**. It is mainly used as a treatment to reduce secretion volumes from the mouth (salivary glands) and respiratory tract. It is used in **children with excessive drooling** and as a premedication agent. Drooling (sialorrhea) is a normal phenomenon in children younger than 18 months but it may persist and become troublesome in children with neurodisability. Estimates of the prevalence of moderate to severe sialorrhea in the developmentally disabled population range from 10% to 40%.

Glycopyrrolate also has some modest sedative and amnesic properties and it **prevents reflex bradycardia**. Less commonly, it can be administered topically to treat hyperhidrosis and can be used to **reverse the neuromuscular blockade** due to non-depolarizing muscle relaxants when it is often co-administered with neostigmine, a cholinesterase inhibitor. It has a longer duration of action than other oral anticholinergics and due to its structure (a quaternary amine) it only poorly crosses the blood–brain barrier. There is an inhaled form (dry powder) that is used in adults in the treatment of chronic obstructive pulmonary disease (COPD). |
Absorption and distribution	Oral glycopyrrolate is **very poorly absorbed** from the gastrointestinal tract. Oral glycopyrrolate has poor bioavailability and a mean of **approximately 3%** is found in the plasma. The tablets are somewhat more bioavailable than liquid formulations in adults and both are significantly less well absorbed in the presence of fat (a reduction of bioavailability of about 75%). If given parenterally the doses required are significantly lower.
Biology	The cation, which is the active moiety of glycopyrronium bromide, is called glycopyrronium or glycopyrrolate. Glycopyrronium blocks **muscarinic receptors** thus inhibiting cholinergic transmission. It reduces the **volume and acidity of gastric secretions** and **controls excessive** oral, pharyngeal, tracheal and bronchial **secretions**. It reduces the rate of salivation by preventing the stimulation of the acetylcholine receptors themselves. It has **widespread activity** on the peripheral parasympathetic system, resulting in predictable dose-dependent biological effects including urinary retention, reduced sweating, increased heart rate, reduced gastrointestinal motility and dilated pupils. It has very limited effects on the central nervous system.
Clearance	Glycopyrronium is largely eliminated unchanged from the renal excretion in urine. It has a biological **half-life** of approximately **3 hours** in adults but data are limited in children. Elimination is severely impaired in children with renal failure and therefore dosing must be reduced.

PRACTICAL PRESCRIBING

Dosing	**For treatment of excessive oral and respiratory secretions** Initial dosing is 20 micrograms (mcg)/kg orally 3 times a day increasing by 20 mcg/kg every 5–7 days based on therapeutic response and adverse reactions. The usual maintenance dose is 40–100 mcg/kg and the maximum recommended dose is 2 mg. **For treatment of hyperhidrosis** Only 1 site to be treated at a time, maximum 2 sites treated in any 24 hours, treatment not to be repeated within 7 days. Treatment of hyperhidrosis requires immersion of the hand or foot in a solution of 0.05% glycopyrrolate and application of a low electrical current. This is a specialized procedure. **As premedication prior to anaesthesia** Neonate: 5 mcg/kg intravenously (IV) or intramuscularly (IM). Child 1 month–11 years: 4–8 mcg/kg (max. dose 200 mcg) IV or IM. Child 12–17 years: 200–400 mcg OR 4–5 mcg/kg (max. dose 400 mcg) IV or IM.
Administration	As fat significantly reduces absorption, glycopyrrolate should be given **at least 1 hour before meals**. Despite widespread use, no oral preparations of glycopyrronium bromide are currently licensed in the UK. The tablets can be crushed and suspended in water and the injectable form can be given orally. Oral formulations, e.g. Sialanar® can be given via a nasogastric or feeding tube but following administration the tube **must be flushed** with 10 mL of water.
Drug errors and safety	Glycopyrrolate reduces sweating ability and can result in **hyperthermia**. Dry mouth, difficulty urinating, headaches, drowsiness, blurred vision, diarrhoea and constipation are all known side effects. As it reduces gastric motility it should be stopped if bowel obstruction is suspected.
Monitoring	The effects of glycopyrronium are monitored clinically and dose adjusted accordingly.
Cost	Glycopyrronium bromide **is fairly expensive**. 1 mg/5 mL oral solution/suspension costs about £3/5 mL. 1 mg and 2 mg tablets cost £8–9 each. Ampoules of injectable glycopyrrolate are very slightly cheaper.

Heparin (unfractionated)

CLINICAL PHARMACOLOGY

Why and when?	Heparin is a naturally occurring polysaccharide released from mast cells. It is used in the **treatment and prevention of thrombotic episodes,** for the maintenance of peripherally and centrally inserted arterial lines, in the maintenance of cardiac and critical stents and in prevention of clotting in extracorporeal circuits. It is also often used as a flush and 'line lock' for central venous catheters (1–6 mL depending on the central line type) in doses of 1–10 units/mL although the evidence for benefit is limited. The concentration is expressed as IU/ mL rather than as a weight due to the variability in its pharmacological action per milligram of drug of product.
Absorption and distribution	Heparin is **not absorbed from the gastrointestinal tract** due to it being a large, negatively charged molecule. Although it can be given via the subcutaneous route, its bioavailability is poor via this route and therefore large doses from this method of administration mean that it is most often given intravenously (IV). It is **highly bound to plasma proteins,** which in part accounts for its variable anticoagulant response following IV administration.
Biology	Heparin is an **indirect inhibitor of the clotting cascade** binding to the naturally occurring antithrombin III (AT) co-factor. Binding to AT causes **inactivation of coagulation factors**, IXa, Xa, XIa, XIIa and thrombin (factor IIa). Heparin binding to AT is reversible, but the AT remains active. Once heparin has dissociated, it can bind to additional AT, providing an ongoing anticoagulant effect. Onset of anticoagulation is extremely rapid. However, it only **prevents further clot formation** and has no effect on an already established clot. It is neither fibrinolytic nor thrombolytic.
Clearance	The **half-life** of heparin is dependent on the route of administration, the dose administered and is subject to wide intra- and inter-individual variability. However, it is **typically around 1 hour**. Clearance is through two independent mechanisms. The first is the saturable binding to proteins, endothelial cells and macrophages, which causes depolarization of heparin. The second is a slower, non-saturable renal clearance.

PRACTICAL PRESCRIBING

Dosing	The dose of heparin is complicated, varies by age and **when available local protocols should be followed**. As guidance, for the treatment of thrombotic episodes, a loading dose of 75 IU/kg is given followed by a continuous IV infusion of approximately 20–25 IU/kg/hour and adjusted according to the activated partial thromboplastin ratio (APTR).

Although unfractionated heparin is rarely used via the subcutaneous route, the dose recommended for the treatment of thrombus is 250 IU/kg twice daily, adjusted according to the APTR, and 100 IU/kg twice daily (max 500 IU per dose) for the prophylaxis of thrombotic episodes, again adjusted according to the APTR. To maintain arterial line patency in neonates the standard dose is 0.5 IU/h with a typical concentration of 1 unit/mL. |
Administration	Unfractionated heparin can be administered subcutaneously but given its low bioavailability via this method of administration it is **mainly used intravenously**. There are multiple concentrations available and care should be taken in selecting the correct product.
Side effects and interactions	As anticoagulation is the desired effect, **haemorrhage** is obviously an important side effect to be aware of. However, due to its relatively short half-life, withdrawal of the drug is usually sufficient treatment. If rapid reversal is required, then **protamine sulfate is a specific antidote**. Other important side effects are heparin-induced thrombocytopenia and hyperkalaemia. Heparin-induced thrombocytopenia is immune mediated and does not usually develop until 5–10 days. If suspected (a reduction in the platelet count of 30% or more) it should be stopped, and an alternative anticoagulant used. Hyperkalaemia is caused by the inhibition of aldosterone secretion, with the risk increasing with the duration of therapy.
Monitoring	The dose of heparin infused is ultimately decided by the **APTR**. Initially the APTR should be taken 4 hours after the start of the infusion and 4 hours after every change in the infusion rate or dose. Local protocols should be consulted for administration of heparin and the dose changes required based on the APTR. In addition to the APTR a baseline **platelet count should be taken before treatment** is started and then **again 4 days later**. Potassium levels should be checked in those at risk of hyperkalaemia, especially if heparin is to continue beyond 7 days. Unfractionated heparin has, in many circumstances (e.g. for use in prevention of further thrombotic events), been supplanted by the use of low molecular weight heparins (LMWH) as these do not require frequent blood testing.
Cost	Unfractionated heparin is **relatively cheap**. Costing depends on the preparation. Flush ampoules for example are around £16 for a pack of 10. Solution for injection ampoules are £15–84 depending on their strength and manufacturer.

Hydrocortisone

CLINICAL PHARMACOLOGY

Why and when?	Hydrocortisone is a corticosteroid with equal glucocorticoid and mineralocorticoid effects. Glucocorticoids have **anti-inflammatory** and **immunosuppressive effects**. It is used orally as a replacement therapy in children with **adrenal suppression** or **insufficiency**. It is also used intravenously in the management of **acute severe asthma, anaphylaxis** and **acute adrenocortical insufficiency** and topically to treat **eczema**. It can also be given acutely for management of hypotension in septic shock if it is unresponsive to inotropes. It is occasionally used rectally for induction of remission in inflammatory bowel conditions such as ulcerative colitis and proctitis if severe and not responding to oral corticosteroids. When used in adrenal insufficiency syndromes, such as **congenital adrenal hyperplasia (CAH)**, hydrocortisone is given with fludrocortisone.
Absorption	Oral hydrocortisone is **readily absorbed** (>95%) via the gastrointestinal tract. It reaches peak concentrations in the plasma by **approximately 1 hour**. Following absorption 90% of hydrocortisone is bound to plasma proteins. Hydrocortisone has poor lipid solubility, therefore in the first 2–3 weeks of neonatal life when bile secretion is poor, it is likely that oral absorption is mildly reduced. Topical hydrocortisone is variably absorbed. Systemic effects are possible, particularly in children with relatively larger surface area to volume ratios and increased skin permeability. The latter is particularly important in newborn and preterm infants.
Biology	Hydrocortisone is an identical molecule to the glucocorticoid hormone cortisol, which is secreted by the **adrenal cortex**. It is essential for regulation of metabolic, cardiovascular and immunological functions. Hydrocortisone release is controlled by a negative feedback mechanism. The hypothalamus secretes corticotrophin-releasing factor (CRF) in response to stress, infection and injury. CRF stimulates the anterior pituitary gland to release adrenocorticotrophic hormone (ACTH), which is released into the circulation to stimulate the adrenal cortex to synthesize and release cortisol. Cortisol release demonstrates **diurnal variation**, typically with an early morning rise. Recent research suggests that outcomes in individuals on long-term replacement therapy are poor due to suppression of the hypothalamic pituitary adrenal (HPA) axis. Therefore, drug regimens that mimic the circadian rhythm of cortisol release within the body are preferred.
Clearance	Hydrocortisone is metabolized by the liver and most tissues to hydrogenated and degraded forms such as tetrahydrocortisone and tetrahydrocortisol. It is then excreted in urine largely in its conjugated form; however, there is a small proportion that remains unchanged. The elimination **half-life** for intravenous or oral hydrocortisone is relatively short at **about 2 hours**, although its duration of action is c.8 hours. Enzyme inducers like phenobarbitone increase the rate of clearance.

PRACTICAL PRESCRIBING

Dosing	In terms of relative glucocorticoid activity 4 mg of hydrocortisone is roughly equivalent to 1 mg of prednisolone, 0.8 mg of methylprednisolone and 150 micrograms of dexamethasone. It has a **shorter half-life** than other commonly used steroids and therefore is **given more frequently**. In severe asthma, IV hydrocortisone dosing is 4 mg/kg every 6 hours. In CAH, oral hydrocortisone is given for all ages at a dose of 9–15 mg/m^2 in 3 divided doses. A slightly lower dose is given for adrenal insufficiency (8–10 mg/m^2 in 3 divided doses). This is often given in conjunction with fludrocortisone. The **smallest possible dose** and the **shortest possible duration** are advised for treatment of skin disorders to prevent systemic adverse effects.
Administration	Intravenous hydrocortisone is administered **over 1–5 minutes** and can be diluted if required with 0.9% sodium chloride, glucose 5% solution or a combination of both. Oral tablets may be crushed or dissolved. When applying topical corticosteroid, it is advised to spread a **thin layer** over the affected areas only and to minimize frequency to once or twice daily. As a suggestion for quantity, **one fingertip unit** (distance from the tip of an adult finger to the first crease delivered from the 0.5 mm nozzle of a tube) is adequate to cover **a surface area twice that of an entire adult hand**.
Drug errors, safety and monitoring	Children who have been on hydrocortisone for long periods of time should have **regular growth monitoring**. Where suspected, suppression of the HPA axis can be confirmed by an ACTH stimulation test. Patients on long-term hydrocortisone therapy are at a significantly increased susceptibility to infection, e.g. chickenpox and shingles due to the immunosuppressive effects of the medication. There are dose-dependent psychiatric side effects associated with prolonged systemic corticosteroid use such as irritability, nightmares and behavioural disturbances. Hydrocortisone tablets should be avoided in those with lactose intolerance as it contains lactose monohydrate. Patients on long-term oral treatment should also be advised to carry 'Steroid treatment' cards to give clear instructions on prescriber, dose, duration and type of steroid they are on.
Cost	Hydrocortisone is **fairly cheap in all forms**. Oral hydrcortisone 10 mg tablets cost around £30 for a pack of 30 tablets. 100 mg of IV hydrocortisone costs just over £1. Some topical hydrocortisone creams and ointments cost less than £1 for 15 g. The most expensive forms are modified-release preparations and enema formulations (foam).
Cream versus ointment	Creams and ointments contain different proportions of oil and water. Ointments have a higher concentration of oil and are therefore greasier and stickier. Creams are easier to spread.

Hyoscine hydrobromide

CLINICAL PHARMACOLOGY

Why and When?	Hyoscine, also known as scopalamine, is a derivative of Belladonna alkaloid. Hyoscine hydrobromide has **central and peripheral anticholinergic activity**. It acts on muscarinic and nicotinic receptors, which are found in the vomiting centres of the brain, and on the salivary glands, smooth muscles and sweat glands. It is used primarily in hospital to treat **excessive salivation** (sialorrhoea) and **smooth muscle spasms**, especially in children with physical disability such as cerebral palsy, or those with poor bulbar control to manage excessive secretions. It is most frequently given via a transdermal patch. It has also been used when a reduction in gastrointestinal secretion and motility is desired, and it is commonly used for the **treatment of motion sickness** due to its central anticholinergic effect on the vomiting centre. It can be purchased in the UK 'over the counter' as Kwells® travel sickness tablets.
Absorption and Distribution	The **bioavailability of oral hyoscine is variable** among individuals ranging from **10–50%. Peak** plasma levels are achieved after **about 30 minutes** and when used for prevention of motion sickness it should be given 30 minutes before travel. The **absolute bioavailability** is somewhat **higher** (c.70%) and a more sustained delivery of hyoscine is achieved when using a **transdermal patch**. With transdermal delivery peak blood levels are reached more slowly, about 6–8 hours after application and there is better maintenance of steady state concentrations and a lower incidence of systemic side effects compared with other anticholinergics as peak concentration side effects are minimised. Unlike the similarly named hyoscine butylbromide (Buscopan®) it **does cross the blood–brain barrier**. It binds reversibly to plasma proteins and binds to skin layers where systemic absorption persists long after the patch is removed.
Biology	As a derivative of Belladonna alkaloid, **hyoscine has anticholinergic effects via competitive inhibition of all five muscarinic receptors**. It also blocks nicotinic receptors at the sympathetic and parasympathetic ganglia. It is widely distributed in the central nervous system (CNS). It inhibits cholinergic impulses from the reticular formation to the vomiting centre. It demonstrates typical symptoms of **parasympathetic blockade**.
Clearance	The elimination **half-life** of an oral dose is **approximately 5 hours**. It undergoes glucuronidation and sulfation in the liver. Less than 10% of the total drug administered is excreted unchanged in urine while the metabolites continue to appear in urine up to and after 100 hours of administration.

PRACTICAL PRESCRIBING

Dosing	The dose of hyoscine is age dependent and varies according to the indication for its use. **None** of the hyoscine preparations available in the UK **are licensed to treat hypersalivation.**
	For motion sickness, children aged **4–9 years** should take **75–150 micrograms orally** 30 minutes before the start of the journey and then **further doses every 6 hours** if required. The maximum daily dose is 450 mcg. Older children and adults can use twice this amount.
	The transdermal patch contains 1.5 mg of hyoscine. It is designed to deliver the drug slowly through intact skin over a period of 72 hours. Although treatment guidelines are based on anecdotal experience children aged **1 month to 3 years should have ¼ patch**, those **3–10 years should have ½ patch** and those **older than 10 years should have 1 patch every 72 hours**.
Administration	Tablets are available in doses of 150 mcg and 300 mcg. The transdermal patch is available as 1.5 mg patches. The transdermal patch should be applied over hairless skin for maximum absorption, preferably behind the ear. The patch **should NOT be cut**. Cutting the patch alters the delivery matrix and impairs drug delivery and absorption. Instead of cutting the patch, an occlusive dressing should be placed on the skin. The fraction of the patch required is placed on bare skin with the remaining fraction resting on the occlusive dressing and covered.
Side effects and interaction	The side effects of hyoscine are mostly due to its anticholinergic effects. Therefore, it may cause **mouth dryness**, increased risk of dental decay, swallowing and speech difficulty, thick and hard to clear secretions, **mucus plugging**, **constipation**, **urinary retention**, sedation, angle closure glaucoma, **blurry vision** and **reduced sweating**. Caution should be taken when used in hot weather. Hyoscine is contraindicated in patients with glaucoma and myasthenia gravis.
Monitoring	No routine monitoring is required but patients should be aware of the side effects and advised to avoid alcohol, driving or operating dangerous machinery whilst on hyoscine.
Cost	Hyoscine is **fairly cheap**. The patches are more expensive than the tablets and annual treatment costs for all patch users are c. £800. A packet of 12 150 mcg tablets costs £1.84 while 12 chewable tablets cost £1.55. Two transdermal patches cost £12.87.

Hypertonic saline

CLINICAL PHARMACOLOGY

Why and when?	Hypertonic saline contains higher molar concentrations of sodium and chloride than 0.9% 'normal' saline. It is **mucoactive**, so can be nebulized to **aid airway clearance in children** with cystic fibrosis (CF) and non-CF bronchiectasis. The osmotic fluid shift resulting from intravenous (IV) administration of hypertonic saline can be used to treat **raised intracranial pressure** or in hyponatraemic seizures.
Absorption and distribution	The distribution of inhaled hypertonic saline is critically **dependent upon the particle size** generated during nebulization. Medium-sized particles (2–4 microM) will land in the conducting airways, with larger particles landing in the mouth, nose and upper airway and therefore not reaching the lungs. When administered intravenously, hypertonic saline immediately enters the circulation, and due to its tonicity (it is hypertonic) it will remain in the circulation.
Biology	Nebulized hypertonic saline exerts mucoactive effects through **multiple modes of action**. Although its primary mode of action is not as a mucolytic, it does **reduce sputum viscosity** by disrupting the ionic bonds in mucus gel and dissociating DNA and mucoprotein. Hypertonic saline is an expectorant as it **increases airway surface water**. This is important in CF as the basic pathophysiology includes increased sodium absorption and decreased chloride secretion, which dehydrates the airway surface and disrupts mucociliary action. Once hypertonic saline is deposited on the airway surface **it draws in additional water through osmosis**. This effect is short lived with airway surface fluid returning to pre-treatment levels within 10 minutes. The water drawn into the airway rehydrates the mucus layer making it easier to clear. Hypertonic saline also **triggers cough**, which increases mucous clearance.
	IV hypertonic saline **increases the vascular osmotic concentration** causing a **shift of fluid** from the intracellular to the intravascular space. This effect is almost immediate. The osmotic shift of fluid reduces raised intracranial pressure. It also **increases cardiac output** due to the volume expanding effects **increasing preload**. Administration of IV hypertonic saline also **increases capillary blood flow**. This occurs due to normalization of endothelial cell volume increasing capillary diameter, reduced plasma viscosity due to increased plasma water content and a direct relaxant effect on vascular smooth muscle.
Clearance	After a bolus of IV hypertonic saline, osmotic equilibrium and therefore cessation of effect are reached after **approximately 4 hours**.

PRACTICAL PRESCRIBING

Dosing	When used to aid airway clearance of mucus the standard regimen is to use **4 mL of 3–7% saline nebulized twice daily**. The concentration used depends, in part, upon side effects. These are experienced variably by individuals and may change over time. In general, **higher concentrations are more likely to cause coughing and bronchoconstriction.**

When used to treat cerebral oedema then either 3% or 2.7% sodium chloride solution may be used. Most emergency regimes suggest using **3 mL/kg of IV 3% sodium chloride over 10–20 minutes**. If possible, central venous access is preferred but it can be given peripherally.

Doses may be repeated. 3 mL/kg increases plasma sodium by approximately 2–3 mmol/L but a greater increase may occur if a large diuresis occurs. For hyponatraemic seizures there is no fixed threshold above which seizures stop, usually an increase in sodium of 3–7 mmol/L is adequate. An acute rise in plasma sodium at a rate less than 10 mmol/L in 24 hours is probably safe. |
Administration	Airway clearance should be **attempted immediately after administration**.
Side effects and interactions	Side effects of nebulized hypertonic saline include coughing, hoarseness and reversible **bronchoconstriction**. These can be reduced by the use of an inhaled bronchodilator prior to administration. Some children report feeling nauseous when higher concentrations are inhaled.
Monitoring	Spirometry should be performed before and after the first nebulized dose to **assess for bronchoconstriction**. When **given IV**, it is sensible to **measure serum electrolytes frequently** to assess the impact and rate of change of serum sodium.
Cost	All preparations of hypertonic saline are **relatively cheap**. 500 mL of 2.7% saline solution for IV use costs c.£4. One month's supply of 7% hypertonic saline for inhalation costs £27.

Tonicity and osmolarity (salt and stuff)

These terms often seem confusing but are relatively simple. The tonicity of a fluid describes the number of solutes present within it that cannot immediately cross a semipermeable membrane. Sodium and chloride ions are examples of solutes that contribute to tonicity. If we add 154 mmol (9 g) of sodium chloride to 1 litre of water then the tonicity is similar to normal serum and therefore described as 'normal saline'. This 0.9% solution is isotonic and isoosmolar. Osmolarity takes into account all of the solute concentrations, not just the ones that cannot cross the semipermeable membrane. Therefore glucose will add to the osmolarity but not the tonicity of a solution. 5% glucose solution has the same osmolality as 0.9% saline but has no tonicity. It is an isoosmolar, hypotonic solution. 5% glucose and 0.45% saline solution is therefore hypotonic and hyperosmolar. **Salt contributes to tonicity. 'Stuff' contributes to osmolarity.**

Ibuprofen

CLINICAL PHARMACOLOGY

Why and when?	Ibuprofen, in its oral form, is one of the most commonly prescribed medications in paediatric practice. Its primary uses are for its **analgesic and antipyretic effects**. Ibuprofen is a non-steroidal anti-inflammatory drug (NSAID), with **anti-inflammatory properties**, so is often used in inflammatory conditions such as juvenile arthritis. Intravenous (IV) preparations can be used in closure of the ductus arteriosus in neonates. It has been shown to be as effective as paracetamol at **improving pain and treating fever**.
Absorption	Ibuprofen is rapidly absorbed from the gastrointestinal tract, with a bioavailability of 80–90%. Ibuprofen has an **onset of action within 30 minutes;** with peak serum levels 1–2 hours following administration. The **effects can last between 6 and 8 hours**, which has been suggested to be longer than that of paracetamol. The anti-inflammatory actions of ibuprofen can take longer, up to 1 week. The bioavailability is minimally altered by the presence of food, which can reduce the rate of absorption but does not decrease the extent of absorption. Conditions which result in delayed gastric emptying may delay the onset of action.
Biology	Ibuprofen is derived from propionic acid and was first introduced in 1969. The main mechanism of action of ibuprofen is by the **non-selective, reversible inhibition of cyclooxygenase enzyme COX-1 and COX-2**. This in turn reduces the production of prostaglandins. Prostaglandins reduce the threshold of pain sensory neurons to stimulation, they are pro-inflammatory, leading to oedema and increased vascular permeability, and they promote leucocyte infiltration.
	Ibuprofen is almost entirely protein bound (98%) and has a low apparent volume of distribution that approximates plasma volume. Unbound concentrations show linear pharmacokinetics at commonly used doses. It is distributed throughout the whole body and can penetrate the central nervous system.
Clearance	Ibuprofen is **rapidly metabolized** in the liver, almost completely, with little or no unchanged drug found in urine. Ibuprofen is primarily metabolized via oxidative pathways involving cytochrome P450 enzymes (preferentially CYP2C9) to two primary inactive metabolites, 2-hydroxyibuprofen and 3-carboxyibuprofen. The excretion is virtually complete 24 hours after last ingestion. The **serum half-life is 1.8–2 hours**. The pharmacokinetic profile of ibuprofen in children appears to be similar to that of adults. Some research suggests that **younger children clear ibuprofen more quickly**.

PRACTICAL PRESCRIBING

Dosing	Age and weight bandings do exist. In practice, most indications require doses of **5–10 mg/kg/dose (to a maximum single dose of 400 mg)** every 6–8 hours. Maximum dosing in a 24-hour period is usually 40 mg/kg/day for pain or fever. Higher doses of 40–60 mg/kg/day can be used in inflammatory conditions to a maximum of 2.4 g per day. The recommended dose for closure of the ductus arteriosus is 10 mg/kg intravenously for 1 day, then 5 mg/kg for 2 days thereafter. This can be repeated after 48 hours if necessary.
Administration	Ibuprofen is most commonly used in the **oral form,** which is easily available for parents to buy over the counter. There are a number of oral preparations available including effervescent granules, modified-release preparations, tablets or capsules (often 200–400 mg per tablet or capsule) and **an oral suspension.** The majority of oral suspensions come in **100 mg/5 mL concentrations**. Ibuprofen can be used topically; however, this is not a route that is often used in children.
Drug errors and safety	Ibuprofen is widely used in paediatrics and **serious toxicity**, even in the case of accidental overdose appears to be **rare in children**. Children may experience symptoms if 100 mg/kg is ingested, and more serious reactions can be seen in doses exceeding 400 mg/kg. In general ibuprofen should be used with caution in children with pre-existing renal, liver or cardiac conditions. Mild gastrointestinal symptoms (nausea or diarrhoea) may occur, especially in longer-term use, but unlike in adults, **significant gastroduodenal pathology is rare**. Abnormal liver function tests, although recognized in children taking ibuprofen, are not often clinically significant. Renal dysfunction is less common in children than adults but is more likely to occur if risk factors exist (dehydration, hypovolaemia, concomitant use of nephrotoxic drugs or renal disease). Ibuprofen has a transient **anti-platelet affect**, which resolves rapidly following doses, which should be considered in children taking other forms of anticoagulation. **NSAID-induced bronchospasm** is less common than in adults. Unless there is a previous history of wheezing on administration ibuprofen can be used, cautiously, in children with asthma.
Monitoring	The majority of children use ibuprofen on a short-term basis and **require no monitoring**. Its effects can be monitored with **response to fever and pain symptoms**. In those children with risk factors, including neonates or those who use ibuprofen in long-term settings **blood monitoring may be recommended.**
Cost	Ibuprofen is **relatively cheap** with a 200 mg tablet costing approx. 6p (brand depending), and the suspension costing 12.5p. IV preparations vary in price and are considerably more expensive.

Insulin

CLINICAL PHARMACOLOGY

Why and when?	Insulin is an endogenous hormone. It is essential to facilitate the transport of glucose into cells and its absence or lack results in diabetic ketoacidosis. In children, it is most commonly used to treat **type 1 diabetes mellitus**. It is less frequently used to treat **cystic fibrosis-related diabetes** mellitus and type 2 diabetes mellitus. Insulin can also be given with glucose infusions to lower serum potassium levels and is used as part of the **emergency management of hyperkalaemia**. Whilst it will lower serum potassium levels, it does not lower total body potassium and other treatments are required to manage potassium overload. There are five **types of insulin analogue available** for use: rapid-acting, regular or short-acting, intermediate-acting, long-acting and ultra-long-acting insulin. Each has different pharmacodynamic properties and understanding these is critical to achieving good glycaemic control.
Absorption	Currently all insulin analogues in the UK **must be given parenterally**. For subcutaneous injections the site plays a small role in determining the precise effects with **abdominal injection** resulting in **quicker absorption**. Absorption is also **delayed if given into areas of lipohypertrophy** and enhanced by local massage or exercise. In the USA an inhaled insulin product is available (Afrezza®). This works within 12–15 minutes and is fully eliminated by 3 hours.
Biology	Endogenous **proinsulin** is mostly secreted by **β-cells in the pancreas**. Proinsulin has some biological effects but these are far less than the cleaved product, insulin, which is about two-thirds the total length (51 amino acids). The last 5 amino acids of insulin are not essential to receptor recognition and binding and substitution of amino acids in this region lead to different biological properties. **Short-acting insulins** are **similar in structure to cleaved insulin**. These will form hexamers *in vivo*, which marginally slow the time to peak activity. **Rapid-acting insulins** have minor modifications in their amino acid sequence that **oppose polymerization**. Long-acting insulins have changes at the terminal end of the insulin molecule (substitutions or additions) and modifications to the protein sequence. These changes **slow absorption** and therefore **prolong the duration of action**.
Clearance	Almost **80%** of endogenous insulin is **removed by the liver**, with a smaller but variable amount cleared by the kidneys and muscles. Clearance rates decrease in obesity, hypertension and liver disease. Fast-acting insulins have an onset of 5–30 minutes, peak at 1 hour and last for 3–5 h. **Regular insulins** have an onset of approximately **1 h**, **peak activity at 2–4 h** and last for **5–8 h**. Intermediate insulin has an onset of 1–2 h, a peak of 4–10 h and a duration of 14 h or more. Long-acting insulins have onset within 4 h, a peak of 6–8 h and a duration of action of up to 24 h. Ultra-long-acting insulin has an onset of action of 1 h, a peak action at 9 h and a duration of action of 36–42 h.

PRACTICAL PRESCRIBING

Dosing	In diabetic ketoacidosis, short-acting insulin infusions should be given at a rate of **0.05–0.1 units/kg/h**. Rates of between 0.02 and 0.125 units/kg/h are need for treatment of hyperglycaemia and neonatal diabetes. Starting subcutaneous insulin doses in children with newly diagnosed type 1 diabetes vary widely from **0.2–0.8 units/kg/day**. Younger children (under 5 years) are at increased risk of hypoglycaemia and children under 5 years are usually started on 0.5 units/kg/day. Older children are usually started on 0.5–0.7 units/kg/day.
Administration	Subcutaneous injection of any medicine is 'a big deal' for most children and families. Insulin is usually administered using a specific device, or '**pen**', which contains **100 units of insulin per millilitre**. The needles are narrow gauge and whilst not pain free, delivery of insulin with a pen device is less painful than delivery with a syringe and separate needle.
	The time to peak effect of short-acting insulin (e.g. Actrapid®) is 2–4 h. **Care therefore must be undertaken before giving further doses**. Elevated blood glucose will take a long time to fully settle, but changes in serum potassium and lactate may be quicker. Local protocols should be followed for insulin infusion. Due to the predictable effects on serum potassium, additional potassium is often added to infusion regimes in diabetic ketoacidosis.
Drug errors and safety	Insulin in overdose is **exceptionally dangerous**. Inconsistencies in prescribing and poor handwriting have led to **avoidable deaths in children**. The word 'units' should be written in full and be clearly separated from any numerals to prevent the 'u' being read as a '0'. The abbreviation IU certainly should be avoided as 5 IU can easily be misread as 51 units. It is exceptionally important to write any insulin prescription very clearly.
Monitoring	Regular **capillary blood gases** and **serum electrolytes** are required for children with diabetic **ketoacidosis**. Blood **glucose and ketone monitoring** is also required for children with diabetes and these should occur **more frequently when unwell**. The glycated haemoglobin (**HbA1c**) gives an indication of longer-term glycaemic control. When insulin is given as a continuous infusion then serum potassium should be measured at least every 4 h.
Cost	Insulin is a **necessary but costly drug**. The NHS spends >£300m per year on insulin in all its forms.

Ipratropium bromide

CLINICAL PHARMACOLOGY

Why and when?	Ipratropium bromide is a drug used in **relieving bronchospasm**, particularly recognized for its use in severe or life-threatening asthma. When used in these circumstances, it should only be used in conjunction with β$_2$-agonists. Less commonly it is also administered intranasally to aid rhinorrhoea in older children. In children with airway **malacia and recurrent wheeze** it is sometimes recommended in preference to salbutamol for acute episodes.
Absorption	When ipratropium bromide is delivered by inhaler or nebulizer, between **10% and 30% of the drug reaches the bronchi** and 7% and 28% of the drug enters circulation within minutes. The remainder of the drug travels into the gastrointestinal tract. Here there is very little absorption that takes place.
Biology	Ipratropium bromide is an **anticholinergic**. When inhaled it is an anti-muscarinic bronchodilator and competitively antagonizes the cholinergic muscarinic receptors (M1, M2, M3) within the bronchial tree. Maximum effects of inhaled ipratropium bromide are seen within 30 and 60 minutes and its duration of action lasts between 3 and 6 hours. In comparison to ipratropium bromide, β$_2$-agonists typically have a quicker onset of action.
Clearance	Once absorbed, ipratropium is excreted via both the kidneys and liver. Ipratropium does not cross the blood–brain barrier. The elimination of ipratropium is biphasic. The **half-life** of elimination of the drug and metabolites is **3–4 h**.

How to give a nasal spray

When giving any medicines via a nasal spray it is important to try to ensure that the delivered medication is not simply swallowed. Therefore **sniffing immediately after administration needs to be discouraged**. It is important that parents and children are taught how to use their sprays and this is re-visited at each review. Nose bleeds are common, particularly if the spray is directed at the nasal septum; this can be minimized by asking the child to use the opposite hand for each nostril (see below).

The steps for most sprays are as follows:

1. **Gently blow your nose** to clear it of mucus.
2. Shake the nasal spray for 10 seconds.
3. Look at your shoes.
4. Holding the spray in your left hand, place it in the right nostril and **spray once whilst gently breathing in through your nose**.
5. Try **not to sniff** for at least 30 sec and continue to breathe **in through your nose but out through your mouth**.
6. Now repeat using the right hand and left nostril.

PRACTICAL PRESCRIBING

Dosing	Age-banded dosing regimens are used. The exact recommended dose depends on indication. The drug delivery is generally much **more efficient** when given via a **valved holding chamber** (spacer) and pressurized metered dose inhaler (**pMDI**), therefore lower doses are required.
	Reversible airways obstruction (by pMDI and spacer): 1 month–5 years – 20 micrograms (mcg) (1 puff) 3 times a day. 6–17 years – 20–40 mcg (1–2 puffs) 3 times a day.
	Acute bronchospasm (by nebulized solution): 1 month–5 years: 125–250 mcg as required (maximum 1 mg/day). 6–11 years – 250 mcg as required (maximum 1 mg/day). 12–17 years –500 mcg as required (maximum 2 mg/day).
	Severe or life-threatening acute asthma (by nebulized solution): 1 month–11 years – 250 mcg every 20–30 min for the first 2 h, then 250 mcg every 4–6 h as required. 12–17 years – 500 mcg every 4–6 h as required.
	Rhinorrhoea associated with allergic and non-allergic rhinitis, by intranasal administration: 12–17 years – 2 sprays 2–3 times a day, dose to be sprayed into each nostril (see over for how to use a nasal spray effectively).
Administration	Inhaled preparations can be given by either **pMDI and spacer** or via **nebulizer**. In life-threatening asthma it can be mixed with salbutamol and nebulized. In these circumstances, nebulizers should be driven by oxygen at 6–8 L/min. At sea level and 20°C a 5 mL volume solution will typically take 6–7 min to be fully nebulized. When given as a nebulizer it is usual practice to dilute the volume to 5 mL with 0.9% saline.
Drug errors and safety	The maximal effect of inhaled ipratropium occurs 30–60 min after administration. Its duration of action will be between 3 and 6 h. Under most circumstances children can be maintained with a treatment schedule of up to 3 times a day. Whilst oral and gastrointestinal absorption are limited it can have local effects and result in a **dry mouth**. Systemic effects include rare cases of urinary retention. Ipratropium given by nebulizer, if misdirected, can deposit in the eye where it results in **pupillary dilation**.
Monitoring	Monitor patients with renal and hepatic impairment. In life-threatening asthma it is important to continuously assess response to treatment.
Cost	Ipratropium is **cheap**. 250 mcg/1 mL nebulizer liquid vials are 24 p each and 500 mcg/2 mL vials are even cheaper. Even the nasal spray is inexpensive, costing about £4 for a month's supply.

Iron (ferrous sulfate, ferrous fumarate, sodium feredetate)

CLINICAL PHARMACOLOGY

Why and when	Iron supplementation may be given **as prophylaxis**, in those **with low stores**, e.g. preterm neonates, children with malabsorption, poor diet, menorrhagia or receiving haemodialysis. It may also be given to treat **iron deficiency anaemia**. This may occur as a consequence of **dietary deficiency** or secondary to other diseases (for example coeliac disease, inflammatory bowel disease or cow's milk protein-induced colitis). Dietary iron may be found in meat, in which it is generally present as haem, of which approximately 20–40% is available for enteric absorption. Non-haem iron in foods such as cereal or spinach is mainly in the ferric state, which needs to be converted to a ferrous form for absorption.
Absorption and distribution	Iron absorption takes place mostly in the **duodenum and upper jejunum**. It is a two-stage process involving first a rapid uptake across the brush border, and then transfer into the plasma from the interior of the epithelial cells. Haem iron is absorbed as intact haem, and the enzyme haem oxidase releases the iron within the mucosal cell; it is then carried in the plasma bound to transferrin. **Non-haem iron is absorbed in the ferrous state** – within the cell, ferrous iron is oxidized to ferric iron, which is then bound to a transferrin-like intracellular carrier. This iron is then either held within the cell as ferritin when the body stores of iron are high, or passed on to the plasma if iron stores are low (where it is then bound to transferrin). **Ascorbic acid can enhance iron absorption** by forming soluble iron-ascorbate chelates and also by reducing ferric iron to the more soluble ferrous form. Certain medications, as well as certain elements in food (such as **tannins** and plant compounds such as **phytic acid**), can also **decrease iron absorption**. A typical presentation of iron deficiency is in the toddler that takes excessive milk, at the expense of a varied diet. Cow's milk (whole milk) has low iron levels and also there is inhibition of non-haem iron absorption by calcium and casein.
Biology	Iron supplementation may be given in the form of several different iron salts, including ferrous fumarate, ferrous sulfate, ferrous gluconate and sodium feredetate. Different forms contain **different amounts of ferrous iron**; there are only marginal differences between these in terms of efficiency of absorption of iron, and haemoglobin regeneration rate is little affected by the type of salt used (provided sufficient iron is given). Most of the iron in the body is present as haemoglobin or myoglobin (75%). The remainder is present in the storage forms soluble ferritin or insoluble haemosiderin, in the reticuloendothelial system, with smaller amounts occurring in haem-containing enzymes (such as cytochromes, catalases or peroxidases) or in plasma bound to transferrin.
Clearance	Ferrous fumarate, ferrous sulfate and sodium feredetate have the same pattern of elimination as dietary iron, which is lost from the body through loss of cells in urine, faeces, hair, skin, sputum, nails and mucosal cells, as well as through blood loss. **There is no active excretion** of iron. A total of approximately 1 mg is lost daily. In children either with iron overload or at risk from it then chelation therapy may be required.

Iron (ferrous sulfate, ferrous fumarate, sodium feredetate)

PRACTICAL PRESCRIBING

Dosing	The oral dose of elemental iron required **to treat deficiency** is **3–6 mg/kg** (max. 200 mg) daily given in 2–3 divided doses. Ferrous fumarate 200 mg contains approx. 65 mg of ferrous iron; ferrous gluconate 300 mg contains 35 mg; and ferrous sulfate 300 mg contains 60 mg. Sodium feredetate (Sytron) is a more common formulation for preterm infants and young children; 190 mg of this contains 27.5 mg of ferrous iron. Duration of treatment should generally not exceed 3 months after correction of anaemia. Co-existing deficiency of vitamin B_{12} or folic acid should be ruled out since combined deficiency can occur.
Side effects and considerations	Common side effects are predominantly gastrointestinal, including **constipation**, abdominal pain, **dark stools** and **diarrhoea**. Dental caries may present an additional risk as forms of sugar are common excipients. There may also be temporary staining of teeth with liquid preparations. **Acute iron toxicity may be fatal**, causing haematemesis (due to corrosive damage of the gastrointestinal mucosa), metabolic acidosis, and haemodynamic instability. It is a particular risk in children as iron-containing tablets may resemble sweets and may be consumed in large quantities.
Monitoring	Monitoring may not be required in the case of iron supplementation for prophylaxis, unless there are clinical concerns. **In iron deficiency, a repeat full blood count after 1 month of iron therapy** at a dose of 3–6 mg/kg daily should show an increase in haemoglobin by at least 1 g/dL. This can be repeated every 2–3 months until the expected normalization has been demonstrated.
Cost	Iron salts are available as oral solutions, oral drops, tablets and capsules. The majority of these are available in generic form, and the **cost of treatment is often low**, with 200 mL of ferrous fumarate 140 mg/5 mL solution costing £3.92, or a packet of 28 tablets of ferrous sulfate 200 mg costing £1.08. However, tablets and capsules may not be acceptable for younger children and sodium feredetate is more commonly prescribed in infants and young children, but is more expensive than other forms. A 500 mL bottle of 190 mg/5 mL oral solution costs £14.95 so on a daily dose of 2.5 mL, this would equate to £0.07 per day but once open the bottle has a shelf life of only 3 months, making this a less cost-effective option.

Isoniazid

CLINICAL PHARMACOLOGY

Why and when?	Isoniazid is a **bactericidal agent** used in the **treatment of tuberculosis (TB)**. It also helps **prevent the development of resistance** in companion drugs. First synthesized in 1912, its anti-tubercular activity was confirmed in the 1950s in clinical trials. It formed part of 'triple therapy' with para-aminosalicylic acid and streptomycin. It has a narrow spectrum of activity being only active against organisms of the genus Mycobacterium, e.g. *M. tuberculosis*, *M. bovis* and *M. kansasii*. It is used as a first-line agent for primary treatment of TB with rifampicin, pyrazinamide and ethambutol. It is used for prophylactic treatment of latent TB either alone or combined with rifampicin.
Absorption and distribution	Isoniazid is **rapidly and almost completely (c.90%) absorbed** after oral administration. Peak serum concentrations occur 0.5–2 hours after an oral dose. It is widely distributed in tissues and body fluids including cerebrospinal fluid (CSF) and breast milk with a volume of distribution ranging from 0.6 to 1.2 L/kg. Oral absorption may be delayed or reduced by food and antacids. It has a low protein binding of <10%.
Biology	Isoniazid is a synthetic derivative of nicotinic acid. It is a **prodrug** and needs activation by a bacterial catalase-peroxidase enzyme called *katG*. It inhibits the synthesis of mycolic acid, required for mycobacterial cell wall. At therapeutic levels isoniazid is **bactericidal against actively growing** intracellular and extracellular *Mycobacterium tuberculosis* organisms; however, it is **bacteriostatic for 'resting' bacilli**. There is a high and growing incidence **of drug resistance** with isoniazid. Approximately 12% of paediatric TB cases worldwide now report isoniazid-resistant TB. Most of the resistance is due to loss of *katG*-encoded catalase peroxidase. However, multiple additional genes are involved in isoniazid resistance. Primary resistance is more prevalent in developing countries.
Clearance	Isoniazid is metabolized primarily by acetylation in the liver, which is genetically determined and differs among various ethnic groups. **Fast acetylators** metabolize the drug 5 times as rapidly as **slow acetylators**. Approximately 50% of Caucasians and Afro-Caribbean are fast acetylators; while 80–90% of Asians and Inuit are slow acetylators. Hence elimination half-life varies from 1 to 1.8 hours in fast acetylators to 3–4 hours in slow acetylators. About 75–90% of the dose is excreted in urine as unchanged drug or metabolites within 24 hours of administration.

PRACTICAL PRESCRIBING

Dosing	Isoniazid dosing in children is **weight dependent**. Dosage for treatment and prophylaxis of TB is **10 mg/kg daily once a day** with a **maximum daily dose of 300 mg per day**. In intermittent supervised regimens, it is used in dosages of 15 mg/kg thrice a week for 6 months. Treatment duration is longer in cases of tuberculous meningitis.
Administration	Isoniazid is dispensed as an injection, liquid or tablet form. Isoniazid should be given on **empty stomach** when administered orally either 30–60 minutes prior or 2 hours after a meal. It is **usually given in the morning**. Tablets should be swallowed with a glass of water, milk or juice and not chewed. Tablets can be crushed and mixed with a small amount of food. Liquid formulations can be measured with a syringe or medicine spoon. Missed doses should be taken as soon as possible, as long as this does is 12 hours before the next dose is due.
Drug errors and safety	Isoniazid may cause **peripheral neuropathy.** In children at increased risk this requires daily supplementation with pyridoxine to prevent it. High-risk children include those with HIV infection, nutritional deficiency and diabetes. Asymptomatic elevation of liver enzymes occurs in 10–20% but it can rarely cause **severe and fulminant hepatitis**, usually within first 3 months of start of treatment. The risk of developing hepatitis is age-dependent (less than 1/1000 for persons younger than 20 years of age). If liver enzymes are raised above 3 times normal levels, isoniazid discontinuation should be considered until levels return to normal and re-start again with small and gradually increasing doses. It is **contraindicated in drug-induced liver disease.**
Monitoring	Routine blood monitoring of isoniazid is **not required**. Monthly liver function tests may be necessary in children with abnormal baseline liver function tests or known liver disease.
Cost	Isoniazid is a **fairly expensive** drug. In tablet form, which is the most common usage, each 100 mg tablet costs around 70p per tablet. Since it is used in a long-term regimens, the overall cost becomes much higher. The IV, which is rarely used, costs around £362 for a 500 mg dose.

Current treatment of tuberculosis in the UK

Tuberculosis is treated in two phases – an **initial phase using 4 drugs** and a **continuation phase using 2 drugs in fully sensitive cases**. Current UK regimens include treatment with rifampicin, isoniazid, pyrazinamide and ethambutol for 2 months followed by 4 months of rifampicin and isoniazid, often combined in a single tablet (Rifater®), which improves adherence.

Ketamine

CLINICAL PHARMACOLOGY

Why and when?	Ketamine is a dissociative **anaesthetic agent**, which is most frequently used in children for sedation and induction of anaesthesia. It also has some secondary **analgesic and amnesic effects.** It should be used only by those with experience in airway management and prior experience of using this class of drug. It induces marked analgesic and hypnotic effect, with patients often described as being in a trance-like state. It is a popular sedative agent as it generally causes very little respiratory depression, maintains airway reflexes and usually increases the blood pressure.
Absorption and distribution	Ketamine is predominantly administered intravenously in paediatric practice, where it has a bioavailability of 100%. Ketamine has **high lipid solubility** but has a low protein binding. This enables **rapid transfer over the blood–brain barrier** (within a minute) and central nervous system (**CNS) levels are typically 4–5 times those seen in plasma**. Ketamine's effects lessen as it is then redistributed to other tissues. If given intramuscularly (IM), bioavailability is high (>90%) and effects are seen within 15–30 minutes but oral bioavailability is much lower (<20%) due to extensive first-pass metabolism.
Biology	Ketamine's anaesthetic effects are exerted through its **antagonistic effect on** N-methyl-D-aspartate (**NMDA) receptors**. These receptors are found at the spinal, thalamic, limbic and cortical level. Ketamine interferes with sensory inputs such as emotion, memory and pain, with EEG studies demonstrating that it causes dissociation between the electrical activity of the thalamus and limbic system. Ketamine is also an analgesic. It is an **opioid receptor agonist**. There are effects on numerous other receptor systems such as agonistic effects of α- and β- adrenergic receptors and antagonistic effect on muscarinic receptors within the CNS. Its action on α-adrenergic receptors results in an **increase in systemic vascular resistance**, which tends to slightly increase blood pressure. Its β-adrenergic effects result in **bronchodilation and tachycardia**.
Clearance	Elimination is via liver metabolism, where ketamine undergoes N-demethylation to norketamine, an active metabolite of ketamine with about 25–30% potency of ketamine. Norketamine undergoes hydroxylation and conjugation in the liver before being excreted renally. The **elimination half-life ranges from 100 to 200 minutes**.

Practice point — Ketamine should only be administered by, or under the direct supervision of, those trained in its use who possess experience of airway management and where resuscitation equipment is readily available.

PRACTICAL PRESCRIBING

Dosing	Dosing is dependent upon a patient's age, weight and hepatic function. The standard dose for children from neonate to 11 years old is **1–2 mg/kg**, titrated according to response. Doses for children 12–17 years of age are given a dosing range of **1–4.5 mg/kg**, titrated to response. Most children require 2 mg/kg. These regimens provide about **5–10 minutes of surgical anaesthesia**. Dosing should be decreased in those with liver dysfunction.
Administration	Ketamine is mainly administered intravenously in paediatric practice. It should be injected over at least 60 seconds. Ketamine is available in 10 mg/mL and 50 mg/mL preparations and these **can be given without dilution**. If an infusion is required for maintenance of anaesthesia then 5% glucose or 0.9% sodium chloride solutions are suitable diluents.
Side effects and interactions	Ketamine is **contraindicated** in children with head trauma, hypertension, raised intracranial pressure, severe cardiac disease and stroke. Caution should be exercised in children with cardiovascular disease, dehydration and intracranial masses. It can (in around 1% of cases) cause laryngospasm, particularly in children with excessive respiratory tract secretions. Users should be **prepared and able to perform a rapid sequence induction** if necessary.
	Other common side effects include mild agitation (20%), moderate/severe agitation (1.5%), rash (10%), vomiting (7%) and transient clonic movements (5%). **Visual hallucinations** are incredibly common in adults and older children.
	Emergence reactions are quite common in children given ketamine for sedation. Children awake with confusion, agitation and hallucinations. These reactions can be minimized with simultaneous use of a benzodiazepine in small doses.
	Ketamine does have some negative inotropic effects, though these are usually offset by its indirect sympathomimetic activity leading to an increase in heart rate and cardiac output. Despite this, ketamine use may lead to **cardiovascular instability in patients with poor cardiac output**, **hypovolaemia** or **low circulating endogenous catecholamines**. As such ketamine should be used with caution in children who have cardiovascular instability or who are on drugs that cause hypotension. Concomitant use of CNS depressing drugs should also be avoided.
Monitoring	Patients receiving ketamine **require cardiovascular monitoring** (heart rate, blood pressure, ECG) and **respiratory monitoring** (respiratory rate and oxygen saturations). Drug levels are not routinely used.
Cost	Ketamine is **relatively inexpensive**. 200 mg of ketamine (as 10 mg/mL) costs just over £5 and 500 mg (as 50 mg/mL) costs around £9 to the NHS.

Lactulose

CLINICAL PHARMACOLOGY

Why and when?	Lactulose is most frequently used to **treat constipation** – it is most useful when used alongside conservative measures such as dietary intervention and behavioural change. It features on the NICE guideline for constipation in children in young people but is not the first-line pharmacological intervention. It can be bought over the counter for use in people over the age of 6; for children under the age of 6 years it can be prescribed. It is also be used in hepatic encephalopathy and small bowel bacterial overgrowth. This use is unlicensed in children but widely used in adult populations.
Absorption	Lactulose itself is **not absorbed into the circulation**. Its effects are predominantly **intraluminal**. It is given as a syrup which typically is made up of roughly two-thirds lactulose together with smaller amounts of galactose (10 g/100 mL), lactose (7 g/100 mL) and fructose (0.6 g/100 mL). **These extra sugars are absorbed.**
	It should therefore be avoided or used with caution in children with lactose intolerance or other disorders of carbohydrate metabolism (such as galactosaemia) and in acute inflammatory bowel disease or bowel obstruction. As the syrup contains significant amounts of sugar it should be used with caution in children at high risk of dental caries or those with diabetes mellitus.
Biology	Lactulose is an **osmotic laxative**. It is a disaccharide molecule composed of fructose and galactose. This stays in the digestive bolus within the gastrointestinal lumen and remains unchanged through the small bowel. In the colon it has a **prebiotic effect**. It is fermented by gut flora and the metabolites (including lactate and acetate) have osmotic properties that draw water into the stool to soften it, making it easier to pass. This metabolism by the colonic flora reduces the pH in the colon, which promotes peristalsis – encouraging passage of stool along the colon.
	The metabolites also **alter ammonia balance** in the gut lumen and effectively reduce the plasma ammonia level, which explains why lactulose is useful in hepatic encephalopathy.
Clearance	Lactulose is **metabolized by colonic flora**. At high doses an amount of unaltered lactulose will pass into the stool.

PRACTICAL PRESCRIBING

Dosing	For constipation: it is most common to use 3.1 g/5 mL or 3.7 g/5 mL solution. In infants less than 1 year 2.5 mL twice daily is the usual starting dose. In children up to 4 years 2.5–10 mL twice daily is used and in older children 5–15 mL twice daily can be used initially. An effect is usually seen after 48 hours. **The dose and frequency can be adjusted to response**. Most paediatricians state that the aim of treatment is to achieve two or three soft stools per day; this definition and aim should be personalized to the child and family, with ease of passage of stool more important than frequency of defecation.
Administration	Lactulose is a sweet-tasting syrup. The liquid can be diluted with water or fruit juice if the taste is unfavourable. It can be taken with or without food, but this may alter the side effect profile (see below). It has a shelf-life of 3 years and should not be stored above 25°C. **Brushing of teeth should be advised after dosing.**
Drug errors and safety	Lactulose is generally well tolerated; common side effects include **bloating, flatulence** (a result of the methane produced by colonic fermentation of the drug), **stomach pain** and **nausea or vomiting**. These usually abate after 1 week. Bloating can be minimized by taking lactulose separately from food and nausea can be minimized by taking lactulose alongside food. Serious side effects such as severe diarrhoea and vomiting, weakness or muscle cramps or an irregular heart rate are much rarer and the drug should be stopped if these occur. Overdose is generally safe, but can cause uncomfortable bloating, flatulence, diarrhoea and nausea. There is a risk of diarrhoea and consequent dehydration with electrolyte (particularly magnesium) depletion.
Monitoring	The drug dose and frequency should be titrated to response. Use alongside a stimulant laxative is often required.
Cost	Lactulose **is inexpensive**. It costs roughly £2.50 for 300–500 mL. Sachets of 'sugar-free' lactulose may be cheaper.

Lamotrigine

CLINICAL PHARMACOLOGY

Why and when?

Lamotrigine is an **antiepileptic drug** (AED). It is a member of the sodium channel blocking class of AEDs. These **suppress the release of glutamate and aspartate**, two of the dominant excitatory neurotransmitters in the central nervous system (CNS). Lamotrigine can also help to prevent low mood (depression) in adults with bipolar disorder. Since its market authorization over 2 decades ago, it is now being used increasingly for the treatment of paediatric epilepsy, becoming the more commonly prescribed new generation AED, especially in young females who may be considering pregnancy in the future. In the UK, lamotrigine is recommended as **monotherapy** for newly diagnosed **focal seizures** and as an **adjunct** for **refractory focal seizures** in children. It is a **second-line** for new-onset **generalized seizures** and a useful **adjunct** for **refractory generalized seizures**. It is the third drug of choice, after ethosuximide and valproate, for absence seizures and it may be administered as a monotherapy or polytherapy.

Absorption

Lamotrigine is **rapidly and almost completely (98%) absorbed** with negligible first-pass metabolism. Its oral bioavailability is 98% and it is not affected by food intake. It is approximately 55% bound to plasma proteins and despite its physicochemical properties (which would suggest poor membrane solubility) it **readily crosses the blood–brain barrier**, possibly through specific transporters.

Biology

The mechanism of action of lamotrigine is related to **inactivation of voltage-dependent sodium channels**. However, this would not account for its apparent action against absence and myoclonic seizures. It may **selectively influence neurons that synthesize glutamate and aspartate**, since it diminishes the release of these excitatory neurotransmitters through its effect on sodium channels.

Clearance

Lamotrigine is metabolized predominantly by **glucuronic acid conjugation in the liver**. Its major metabolite is an inactive 2-n-glucuronide conjugate. Metabolites are renally excreted with less than 10% of the drug excreted unchanged. Caution is advised in renal failure as metabolites may accumulate. The **half-life is around 24–35 hours** in all ages. However, when used concomitantly with enzyme-inducing drugs, the **half-life is reduced** to approximately **14 h**, and, **in the presence of valproate, increased to about 70 h**. A steady state is reached after 3–15 days, depending on whether it is taken with enzyme-inducing drugs, valproate or neither. The dosing of lamotrigine in children on adjunctive therapy is highly dependent on the effect of the co-administered drugs. Higher doses are required when it is used with 'enzyme-inducing' AEDs, such as phenobarbital, phenytoin, carbamazepine and oxcarbazepine. Conversely, valproate reduces clearance and raises the plasma concentration by as much as two-fold; hence, a lower dose is recommended. Co-administration with valproate has also been found to increase lamotrigine's most serious side effect of severe rash (**Stevens–Johnson syndrome**).

PRACTICAL PRESCRIBING

Dosing	For oral administration, lamotrigine is licensed from 12 years onwards for monotherapy. It is introduced at a dose of **25 mg once daily for 14 days**, then increased to 50 mg once daily for a further 14 days. Increases of up to 100 mg every 7–14 days are then used to a **usual maintenance dose of 100–200 mg daily in 1–2 divided doses**. It can be increased if necessary up to 500 mg daily.
	When used as an adjunct therapy in those already taking valproate, smaller initial doses are used. For example, as above, in children 12 years and over, the initial dose should be **25 mg once daily on alternate days for 14 days**, then 25 mg once daily for further 14 days. This is then increased in steps of up to 50 mg every 7–14 days with a maintenance dose of **100–200 mg daily in 1–2 divided doses**.
	In those already taking enzyme-inducing drugs, larger initial doses are needed. In children >12 years the initial dose should **be 50 mg once daily for 14 days**, then 50 mg twice daily for further 14 days. This is increased in steps of up to 100 mg every 7–14 days to a **maintenance dose of 200–400 mg daily in 2 divided doses**, up to 700 mg daily if needed.
Side effects and considerations	Lamotrigine poses the **risk of Stevens–Johnson syndrome**. The risk peaks at around 2 weeks after initiation of treatment and diminishes after 8 weeks. The risk is highest in children, when there is a higher starting dose, with a quicker titration of dose and when it is co-administered with valproate. **Lamotrigine should always be introduced gradually**. Other common side effects include dizziness, sleepiness, double vision and nausea. A benign rash occurs in up to 10% of patients. Children's skin may **become more sensitive to sunlight**. When outdoors, they should wear a long-sleeved top, trousers and a hat, and should wear a high-factor sunscreen (SPF 30+). They may develop a tremor; their coordination can be affected, or they may develop blurred vision. They can have changes in mood, may be aggressive or hyperactive, and some have sleep disturbance or sleep initiation problems.
	In pregnancy caution is advised, but the benefits of the medication may outweigh the potential risks. So far there is no indication that lamotrigine causes serious birth defects, but there have been no well-controlled studies in women, and studies in animals have shown some harm to the fetus. It is secreted in breastmilk, but limited data suggest no harmful effect on infants.
	Treatment should not be discontinued abruptly as seizures may be precipitated. It should be tapered over a period of 5–6 weeks. Care should be taken when switching between oral formulations in the treatment of epilepsy. Patient information for parents is available at https://www.medicinesforchildren.org.uk/lamotrigine-preventing-seizures.
Cost	Lamotrigine **is inexpensive**. It is available as an oral suspension, oral solution, tablet and dispersible tablet. The treatment cost is low with dispersible tablets in packs of 30 tablets costing between £2 and £4 per pack. At usual doses it **costs around £4 per month** when used as monotherapy.

Levetiracetam

CLINICAL PHARMACOLOGY

Why and when?	Levetiracetam is used **to treat epilepsy**. It is a member of the second-generation antiepileptic drugs (AEDs). It is relatively new and has been available since 2000. It was developed as an analogue of piracetam, a drug used to improve cognitive function, and was discovered by accident to have antiepileptic activity in animal models. Its advantages include rapid and almost complete absorption, minimal insignificant binding to plasma protein, absence of enzyme induction, absence of interactions with other drugs and partial metabolism outside the liver. It is effective for both partial and generalized seizures, is relatively well tolerated and appears not to interact with other drugs. It is starting to become the first choice of antiepileptic in focal seizures and myoclonic seizures.
	It has been used intravenously in **acute treatment of status epilepticus in children** in place of phenytoin, where its effectiveness appears to be similar. Phenytoin has a less favourable safety profile and is a negative inotrope.
Absorption and distribution	**Levetiracetam** is rapidly absorbed after oral administration, with peak concentration occurring after 1.3 hours, and its bioavailability is >95%. It is only minimally bound to plasma proteins (<10%) and appears to **readily cross the blood–brain barrier**. When given intravenously to children in status epilepticus, the median time to seizure cessation was 35 minutes (compared with 45 minutes for phenytoin). When given orally **co-ingestion of food slows the rate but not the extent of absorption**, reduces the peak plasma concentration by 20% and delays it by 1.5 hours.
Biology	Its mechanism of action remains uncertain but is **distinctly different from other AEDs**. Levetiracetam binds to a protein on the presynaptic neuronal plasma membrane and **modulates release of excitatory neurotransmitters**, such as **glutamate**, by binding to the synaptic vesicle protein SV2A in the brain. It also produces **blockade of voltage-gated N-type Ca2+ channels**.
Clearance	Approximately one-third of a levetiracetam dose is metabolized and two-thirds are excreted in urine unchanged. The **metabolism is not hepatic** but occurs primarily in blood by hydrolysis. Autoinduction is not a feature of its metabolism. The **biological half-life of levetiracetam is 7 hours** and typical oral-dosing regimens are twice daily for established treatment. As clearance is renal in nature it is directly dependent on creatinine clearance. Therefore, dosage adjustments are necessary for patients with moderate-to-severe renal impairment.

PRACTICAL PRESCRIBING

Dosing	Levetiracetam is licensed in Europe for monotherapy **in focal seizures** with or without secondary generalization **in children over the age of 16 years** and as an adjunctive therapy of myoclonic seizures and tonic-clonic seizures.

As monotherapy the starting dose is 250 mg once daily increasing to twice daily after 1-2 weeks and then according to response every 2 weeks (max. 1.5 g twice daily). As adjunctive therapy, the starting dose in children over 6 months of age (body weight up to 50 kg) is 10 mg/kg once daily, which is then increased in steps of up to 10 mg/kg twice daily, every 2 weeks. **The usual treatment dose range is 30–50 mg/kg/day** (max. 60 mg/kg/day) **in 2 divided doses**.

In children over 50 kg the starting dose is 250 mg twice daily, then increased in steps of 500 mg twice daily (max. per dose 1.5 g twice daily), with the dose increased every 2–4 weeks. If switching between oral therapy and intravenous (IV) therapy (for those temporarily unable to take oral medication), the IV dose should be the same as the established oral dose.

When used to treat acute seizures the doses used in research studies **were 40 mg/kg over 5 minutes** (age range 6 months–18 years). |
| Administration | Levetiracetam is available as an oral solution 100 mg/mL and a wide range of oral tablets in sizes 250 mg, 500 mg, 750 mg and 1 g. There are also 250 mg, 500 mg and 1 g granule sachets. There is a 500 mg/5 mL concentrate for IV infusion. |
| Side effects and considerations for use | When starting levetiracetam it should be noted that a child may experience a decreased appetite, nausea and/or vomiting, have stomach ache or diarrhoea. A rash may develop. Headache or dizziness can occur. **Most side effects settle within the first few weeks**.

Behaviour may be affected. Children may be drowsy, less alert than normal and may say they cannot think clearly or remember things. They may develop a tremor, or their coordination may be affected, seeming clumsy. They may also have changes in mood and may be aggressive or hyperactive (more active than usual and finding it hard to relax). A small number of children will develop a severe behavioural change known as **'Keppra rage'**. |
| Cost | Levetiracetam is a **cost-effective AED**, although it is somewhat more expensive than older alternatives. The oral suspension (100 mg/mL) costs around £8 for 100 mL. Granules vary in cost for 60 sachets from £22 to £76 as the dose increases. Tablets are usually the most cost-effective option: typical prices are £3–£9 for a pack of 60. Intravenous preparations are a little more expensive, a 500 mg/5 mL vial costs c.£13. It therefore costs about £1 per kg of bodyweight of the child when used in status epilepticus. |

Levothyroxine sodium

CLINICAL PHARMACOLOGY

Why and when?	Levothyroxine is a synthetic thyroxine (T_4) medication. It is used as a **replacement therapy** in the absence or deficit of thyroid hormones in **hypothyroidism** or as an adjunct with thyroid blocking therapy in hyperthyroidism. It can be used in children of all ages. Neonatal hypothyroidism requires prompt treatment to facilitate normal development. It is available in oral form only. In emergency situations, e.g. hypothyroid coma, where more rapid onset of action is required, liothyronine sodium may be given by intravenous (IV) injection.
Absorption	Absorption can range from 40% to 80%, with most of the drug being absorbed in the jejunum and upper ileum. Levothyroxine has a **relatively slow absorption time** and then rapidly equilibrates in extracellular fluid, meaning that there is little post-ingestion change in circulating concentration. It is transported in the blood bound to thyroxine-binding globulin.
	Antacids, calcium salts, oral **iron,** lanthanum, polystyrene sulfonate and sucralfate are all documented to **decrease absorption of levothyroxine** and so separating administration by 2–4 hours is recommended.
Biology	Levothyroxine works as a **synthetic free-T_4,** which is then converted to liothyronine (T_3) upon entry to the cells. T_3 has a high affinity for nuclear thyroid hormone receptors.
	Thyroid hormones produce a **general increase in the metabolism** of carbohydrates, fats and proteins in most tissues. This, along with the effects of other hormones in the body, brings about an **increase in the basal metabolic rate**, which produces an increased oxygen consumption and heat production. Levothyroxine requirements can increase during pregnancy. It may cross the placenta and excessive or insufficient maternal thyroid hormones can be detrimental to the fetus.
Clearance	The liver is the major site of metabolism with the free and conjugated forms excreted partly in the bile and partly in the urine. The **half-life of thyroxine in the hypothyroid state is 9–10 days,** meaning that (along with the slow absorption) there is little variation of circulating concentration following administration or with varying times of ingestion.

PRACTICAL PRESCRIBING

Dosing	Dosing is dependent on age and is **changed according to serum thyroid stimulating hormone (TSH) and T$_4$ levels** as well as **symptoms**. Neonatal doses start at 10–15 micrograms/kg once daily and are adjusted in steps of 5 mcg/kg every 2 weeks until an optimum dose is found. Children 1 month–1 year of age should start on 5 mcg/kg once daily, which should be adjusted every 2–4 weeks. Children 2–17 years of age should start at a dose of 50 mcg once daily, which should be adjusted in steps of 25 mcg every 2–4 weeks (2–11 years) and 25–50 mcg every 2–4 weeks in older children (12–17 years).
Administration	Levothyroxine is available in tablet, oral solution and capsule form. Tablets of 12.5, 25, 50, 75 and 100 mcg are available. Capsules are also available in 25, 50 and 100 mcg strengths. Solutions are available for younger children and come in 5 mcg/mL, 10 mcg/mL and 20 mcg/mL. Levothyroxine should be taken at the same time each day, preferably 30 minutes before meals, caffeine-containing drinks or other medication.
Drug errors and safety	As levothyroxine is a synthetic hormone its side effects are usually found with excessive doses (i.e. thyrotoxicosis). These include heat intolerance, weight loss, tachycardia, hypertension, diarrhoea, vomiting, muscular atrophy, weakness, thin skin and exophthalmos. In this instance medication may be stopped for a short period of time before being recommenced at a lower dose. **Due to there being three different strengths of oral solution, care should be taken to avoid medication errors; make sure the same strength is specified.** Prescribers should also be cautious when prescribing with cardiac disorders, starting at a low dose and titrating up.
Monitoring	Monitoring should initially be done **every 2 weeks** after commencing therapy to find a therapeutic range. After this, less frequent monitoring is required to ensure that no changes need to be made to the dose. It is important to note that more frequent testing may be required in certain circumstances (such as pregnancy). In most cases (c.90%) of congenital **hypothyroidism** the central component of thyroid regulation remains intact and therefore **TSH monitoring alone will usually be sufficient**. Low TSH suggests excess and high TSH suggests insufficient dosing or diminished adherence to therapy. As the half-life is long, **a single missed dose on the morning of testing should not significantly increase TSH levels**. In central hypothyroidism, free T$_3$ and T$_4$ also need to be measured.
Cost	Levothyroxine in tablet form is **relatively cheap** with 28 tablets costing £4–15. The oral solution is more expensive with 100 mL of 25 mcg/5 mL costing approximately £95.

Lidocaine

CLINICAL PHARMACOLOGY

Why and when?	Lidocaine, also known as lignocaine, is a local anaesthetic agent. It may be injected or applied topically to the skin as **EMLA® cream** to minimize the discomfort of procedures such as venepuncture. Injectable lidocaine solution is frequently used for **infiltration anaesthesia** and for performing peripheral and regional **nerve blocks**. Lidocaine is also formulated as a spray (**Xylocaine®**) that can be applied to the mucosal membranes of children. This reduces the risk of **laryngospasm** during general anaesthesia and endoscopic procedures. Lidocaine is often the first-choice of local anaesthetic in children when a **rapid onset of action** and **intermediate duration of effect** are required. Lidocaine is also a **Class Ib anti-arrhythmic** agent that is used uncommonly in children for ventricular arrhythmias and pulseless VT. Intravenous lidocaine may be considered as an alternative to amiodarone when the latter is unavailable or contra-indicated.
Absorption and distribution	After infiltration, the onset of the local anaesthetic effect of lidocaine is **around 1–5 minutes**, and up to 15 minutes after a peripheral nerve block. The speed of onset and efficacy appear to be **slower and reduced in inflammation** and acidosis. EMLA® cream has maximum effects at 60–90 minutes. Lidocaine is lipid-soluble. The duration of clinical effects when used as a local anaesthetic depends upon its local clearance by systemic absorption. This is related to dose, local blood flow and local tissue binding. The addition of **epinephrine** to lidocaine solution slows systemic absorption and prolongs its local effects.
Biology	Lidocaine belongs to the **amide class of local anaesthetics**. These are less likely to produce an allergic reaction than esters. Lidocaine reversibly binds to the voltage-gated sodium channels of the axon membrane to prevent them from opening. As a result, **the transient influx of sodium into the nerve cell is blocked** and there is no subsequent generation and propagation of the action potential along the axon. When used intravenously as an antiarrhythmic agent, lignocaine acts to shorten the duration of the cardiac action potential, slow conduction velocity and increase the length of the refractory period.
Clearance	The vast majority (>95%) of the drug is ultimately metabolized by the cytochrome **P450 3A4 enzyme** in the liver. Lidocaine has one of the shortest half-lives of the local anaesthetics, at c.**90–110 minutes.** The half-life of lignocaine may be prolonged in patients with hepatic impairment or congestive heart failure.

PRACTICAL PRESCRIBING

Dosing	Lidocaine is commonly available as 1% (10 mg/mL) solution for injection. Solutions are also available with or without epinephrine at 5 micrograms (mcg)/mL (1 : 200,000). For infiltration and regional anaesthesia, infants and children may receive up to 3 mg/kg of the drug. An interval of at least 4 hours must elapse before the dose can be repeated. To avoid excessive dosage in obese patients when used by local infiltration, weight-based doses may need to be calculated on the basis of ideal body weight.
	When applied topically to the skin or mucus membranes, e.g. as EMLA® cream (2.5% lidocaine, 2.5% prilocaine) or Xylocaine® spray (10 mg/dose), the maximum dose of the drug is also determined by the child's weight and age. In neonates, it is important that the maximum dose (1 g) of EMLA cream applied to the skin is not exceeded due to an increased risk of **methaemoglobinemia** in this age group. In order to reduce the risk of toxicity, clinicians should try to **give the lowest dose of the drug necessary to achieve effective local anaesthetic**.
Administration	EMLA cream is usually applied under an occlusive dressing. The **duration of analgesia after removal** of the cream **is around 30–60 minutes**. In many cases, local anaesthetic will be used as an adjunct to general anaesthesia in children. Local anaesthetic alone can be used for minor procedures as long as the child is able to understand what is happening and keep still during the procedure. When administering lignocaine as an injectable local anaesthetic in an awake child, distraction with audio-visual stimuli is an effective means to reduce pain caused during administration. Asking the child to raise their leg during the injection can also provide distraction.
Drugs errors and safety	Lidocaine is generally a very safe drug. However, incorrect dosing, or accidental intravascular injection, may cause **local anaesthetic systemic toxicity (LAST).** Features include generalized seizures, cardiac arrhythmias and arrest. Therefore, **it is imperative that children are accurately weighed before any procedure where local anaesthetic will be used to ensure safe dosage levels are not exceeded**. Whilst injecting a lignocaine solution, it is important to frequently pull back on the plunger to check for blood entering into the syringe, which may indicate inadvertent venous or arterial injection. Additional caution is also required with the use of lignocaine solutions containing adrenaline due to the **risk of ischaemia**. Adrenaline is contraindicated for ring block of digits or the penis.
Monitoring	If the child is awake for a procedure or surgery, then the quality of local anaesthesia may be monitored clinically.
Cost	Lidocaine solution **is cheap**, with an NHS indicative price of around £4.40 per 10 mL-ampoule. EMLA cream is also relatively inexpensive at approximately £2.25 per 5 g.

Low-molecular-weight heparin (LMWH)

CLINICAL PHARMACOLOGY

Why and when?	There are many types of low molecular weight heparin (LMWH) including enoxaparin and tinzaparin, with each one having its own dose, pharmacodynamic and pharmacokinetic properties. In general, their longer half-lives, dose-dependent renal clearance and increased bioavailability from subcutaneous injection mean that they are favoured more than unfractionated heparin. As their name suggests, they have a lower molecular weight than standard heparin, typically around 4000–6500 Da. They are given by the subcutaneous route and used for **the treatment and prophylaxis of thrombotic episodes**.
Absorption and distribution	Due to their lower molecular weight, in comparison to heparin, LMWHs have much higher bioavailability when administered by subcutaneous injection (>90%). They have a much lower affinity for plasma and matrix proteins leading to a **more predictable anticoagulant response**. They have a relatively low volume of distribution and peak anti-Xa activity occurs 3–4 hours after administration.
Biology	Like heparin, LMWHs are indirect inhibitors of the clotting cascade binding to the naturally occurring antithrombin III (AT) cofactor. However, they differ from heparin in that their **main mechanism of action is to inhibit factor Xa**. This is because the chain length of the molecule is not long enough to inhibit the production of factor IIa. They have very little effect on the activated partial thromboplastin ratio (APTR). Like heparin, they only act as an anticoagulant and are not fibrinolytics or thrombolytics.
Clearance	LMWHs are almost exclusively renally cleared, but the half-life varies between the different LMWHs available. In general, their half-lives are **considerably longer than heparin**, which allows once to twice daily dosing. Children, especially those who are younger, appear to clear LMWH more quickly than older children and adults.

PRACTICAL PRESCRIBING

Dosing	The dose of LMWH is specific to the one being prescribed. The dose is not interchangeable (unit for unit) as they differ in their molecular weight, anti-Xa and anti-IIa activity and plasma half-lives. As a general rule, **higher doses** per kg in weight are **required in younger children**, with neonates, for example, requiring up to double the dose of enoxaparin in comparison to a 2-month-old for the treatment of a thrombotic episode (1.5–2 mg/kg twice daily for a neonate, 1.5 mg/kg twice daily for a 1-month-old child, and 1 mg/kg daily for children aged between 2 months and 17 years). Lower doses are used for prophylaxis of thrombotic episodes (750 micrograms (mcg)/kg twice daily of enoxaparin for children <2 months and 500 mcg/kg twice daily for children 2 months and older).

This may be due to a larger volume of distribution, increased clearance and/or lower plasma concentrations of antithrombin III. Unlike adults where the anticoagulation activity is unmonitored, the dose of LMWHs in children is often **guided by an antifactor Xa level**. |
| Administration | LMWHs are administered by **subcutaneous injection**. Pre-filled syringes are available but only go down to a concentration of 20 mg/0.2 mL for enoxaparin. Care should be taken in younger children when small doses are difficult to administer. Sometimes a subcutaneous catheter is inserted to avoid repeated injections in children. If used, the catheter can usually remain *in situ* for several days before being changed. |
| Side effects and interactions | As anticoagulation is the desired effect, haemorrhage is obviously an important side effect to be aware of. If rapid reversal is required then **protamine sulfate** is a specific antidote, although unlike with heparin, it only **partially reverses the effect**. Other important side effects are heparin-induced thrombocytopenia and hyperkalaemia. Heparin-induced thrombocytopenia is immune mediated and does not usually develop until 5–10 days. If suspected (a reduction in the platelet count of 30% or more) it should be stopped, and an alternative anticoagulant used. Hyperkalaemia is caused by the inhibition of aldosterone secretion, with the risk increasing with the duration of therapy.

Unsurprisingly, LMWH's main interactions are with other drugs that act on the clotting cascade. However, there is also an increased risk of bleeding when it is used with some antidepressants, especially the SSRIs. |
| Monitoring | Unlike in adults, **monitoring of antifactor Xa levels is recommended** in children. The target range is 0.5–1 unit/mL. As a guide, levels should be taken 4–6 hours post injection, but where available local protocols should be followed. Like with heparin, platelets and potassium should be monitored due to the risk of heparin-induced thrombocytopenia and hyperkalaemia secondary to inhibited aldosterone secretion. |
| Cost | LMWH is **more expensive than unfractionated heparin**, but the costs for consumables (syringes, infusion sets, syringe drivers) are much lower. The cost depends on the formulation used. Enoxaparin pre-filled syringes vary between £20 and £100 for a pack of 10, depending on strength and manufacturer. |

Magnesium

CLINICAL PHARMACOLOGY

Why and when?

In the paediatric population, magnesium is most commonly used as part of the management of acute **asthma exacerbations** in children older than 2 years. Magnesium use in this instance is second line and given when other interventions such as inhaled or nebulized bronchodilators (such as salbutamol and ipratropium and oral steroids) have not improved symptoms adequately. In children with asthma it can be given intravenously or as a nebulizer. It can also be used in **persistent pulmonary hypertension** of the newborn (PPHN), **hypomagnesaemia**, neonatal hypocalcaemia, constipation, **torsade de pointes**, management of hypertension and seizures associated with eclampsia and treatment of renal tubular diseases or toxicity (e.g. Gitelman syndrome). NICE guidance recommends: 'consider adding magnesium sulfate to nebulized salbutamol and ipratropium bromide in the first hour in children >2 years with a short duration of acute severe asthma symptoms presenting with an oxygen saturation less than 92%'.

Absorption

Magnesium can be taken orally, as a nebulized solution of isotonic magnesium sulfate or intravenously. Oral administration of magnesium is absorbed in the small intestine (especially the ileum) and the colon. **Bioavailability** of magnesium salts from the **oral route is quite poor**, with only around 10–30% being absorbed. Oral magnesium may be encountered in some laxatives or antacids, e.g. Picolax®. When given as a nebulizer or intravenously it has an almost immediate onset of action.

Biology

Magnesium is the fourth most common cation in the body and 40% of magnesium is bound to plasma proteins. An adult has about 24 g of magnesium, of which most is stored in bone (60%), muscle (20%) and soft tissue (20%). Only 2–3% of the total exists in the active, ionized form. Adults and children with **acute asthma have lower intracellular magnesium levels**. Low serum levels are also found in children taking loop or thiazide diuretics.

It is the magnesium cation in magnesium sulfate that is responsible for the bronchodilator effect. It **inhibits calcium release** from endoplasmic reticulum and activates sodium-calcium channel pumps. Calcium is therefore unable to interact with myosin which results in **smooth muscle relaxation**. Magnesium also contributes to T-cell stabilization, stimulation of nitric oxide and prostacyclin synthesis, and inhibition of mast-cell dysregulation and acetylcholine release. It may also potentiate the effects of β_2-agonists by augmenting the β_2-receptor affinity for agonists. These effects lead to a reduction in smooth muscle excitability, further bronchodilation and relief of symptoms.

Clearance

Magnesium has a relatively short **half-life** of **2.5–3 hours**. Magnesium is rapidly renally excreted after administration, mainly from the distal convoluted tubule. Whilst toxicity and retention are rare, renal dysfunction can result in hypermagnesaemia.

PRACTICAL PRESCRIBING

Dosing	For use in acute asthma in children >2 years, magnesium sulfate ($MgSO_4$) is used either as an **intravenous (IV) infusion 40 mg/kg (max 2 g per dose) to be given over 20 minutes** or nebulized as 2.5 mL of isotonic $MgSO_4$. Dosing for IV preparations is by weight, as weight has been shown to affect volume distribution and clearance. For treatment and prevention of hypomagnesaemia oral magnesium aspartate/glycerophosphate can be given, and doses are as per age. **Magnesium hydroxide has a laxative effect** and therefore can be used in constipation; magnesium sodium picosulfate is used for bowel preparation prior to procedures. Magnesium salts are used as antireflux medications.
Administration	Magnesium can be given orally, nebulized or intravenously. In nearly all circumstances it is best to give as IV at a **maximum concentration of 10% solution**. If necessary, it can be diluted with either 5% glucose or 0.9% sodium chloride solutions. **When used as a nebulizer, a total dose of 150 mg in 2.5 mL is required**. This is difficult to achieve precisely using 10% or 50% $MgSO_4$ solution. For example 1.5 mL of 50% $MgSO_4$ solution (750 mg) can be added to 11 mL of 0.9% saline (total volume 12.5 mL) and 2.5 mL of the resulting solution should then be used as a nebulizer. It can be co-administered with other bronchodilators (e.g. salbutamol). Practical difficulties in calculations in emergency situations and unfamiliarity with its use have limited the uptake of nebulized magnesium in the UK.
Drug errors and safety	Magnesium is a **relatively safe drug** when given at the correct doses and rates. Patients being given an IV magnesium infusion should be on a cardiac monitor due to its cardiac effects. Due to its renal excretion those with renal failure should be monitored closely for toxicity. Plasma magnesium levels are normally between 0.75 mmol/L and 0.95 mmol/L; these can rise rapidly (but transiently) when IV or nebulized magnesium is given. Patients with plasma concentrations up to 4 mmol/L often develop **facial flushing** secondary to vasodilation. Higher plasma concentrations cause **hypotension**, loss of deep tendon reflexes, **bradycardia** and potentially respiratory arrest.
Monitoring	Efficacy is assessed by the improvement in the patient's condition. During infusion, heart rate, respiratory rate, **blood pressure** and serum magnesium levels should be monitored closely. Hypermagnesaemia can lead to cardiac arrythmias and PR, QRS and QT abnormalities. Other signs include nausea, vomiting, muscle weakness, muscle paralysis, blurred vision, diplopia and central nervous system (CNS) depression. Magnesium administration is considered safe in pregnancy and breastfeeding.
Cost	Magnesium sulfate is **relatively cheap**. 50% (magnesium 2 mmol/mL) solution for injection 10 mL ampoules (500 mg/1 mL) cost just over £2 each.

Mannitol

CLINICAL PHARMACOLOGY

Why and when?	Mannitol is an osmotic diuretic. It is a naturally occurring sugar alcohol found in fruits and vegetables. It is metabolically inert and is excreted by glomerular filtration. In order for it to have a systemic effect it must be given intravenously. Its effect increases plasma osmolality, which enhances the movement of water from tissues, such as cerebrospinal fluid and the brain into plasma and interstitial fluid, leading to diuresis. As a result, in paediatric practice mannitol is used for **cerebral oedema**, **peripheral oedema** and **ascites**. In all three cases it can be used in children aged 1 month–17 years, although the dosage per kilogram varies depending on age. Studies have also used inhaled mannitol in **asthma** and **cystic fibrosis**. It is available for hospital use in intravenous (IV) forms.
Absorption	Orally it is poorly absorbed from the gastrointestinal system and as a result can cause an osmotic diarrhoea. It is not metabolized within the body and is excreted by glomerular filtration.
Biology	Mannitol **increases the blood osmolality** causing the flow of water from tissues into the plasma and interstitial fluid to increase. It has its effect at the **renal tubules**, in particular its osmotic activity is exerted on the proximal convoluted tubule and the descending limb of the loop of Henle. Its presence within the tubules increases the osmolality of the filtrate, which prevents water from being reabsorbed. Additionally, due to its osmotic effects it resists the action of the antidiuretic hormone (ADH) in the collecting tubule, which prevents passive tubular reabsorption. Correspondingly **it increases urine output**. As well as the increased urine volume, the urine flow rate increases; as a result $Na+$ reabsorption is reduced, which creates a natriuresis. The natriuresis is of a lower magnitude than the water loss, which eventually causes hypernatraemia.

Mannitol does not pass the blood–brain barrier, which causes an osmotic gradient between the brain tissue and plasma. As result fluid from the brain tissues moves towards the plasma, causing a decrease in intracranial pressure (ICP). Plasma expansion also decreases plasma viscosity improving cerebral perfusion and limiting ischaemic damage. |
| Clearance | Mannitol is **not metabolized**, it is excreted unchanged by **glomerular filtration**, without any tubular reabsorption. It has a half-life of approximately **2 hours**, which is significantly increased in renal failure. |

PRACTICAL PRESCRIBING

Dosing	The dosing regimen for mannitol is based on age and weight. Its beneficial effect in **cerebral oedema** is achieved at dosages of **0.25–1.5 g/kg in children 1 month–11 years**, in older children **12–17 years** higher doses of **0.25–2 g/kg** are indicated in order to achieve its clinical effect. In **cerebral oedema** the dosage should be delivered over **30–60 minutes**. The dosing regimen allows the dose to be repeated 1–2 times after 4–8 hours if necessary.

Mannitol has other clinical uses in **peripheral oedema** and **ascites**; in these cases a dosage of **1–2 g/kg** is delivered over **2–6 hours**. In all cases mannitol should be administered preferably by a central vein or a large peripheral vein; doing so reduces the risk of phlebitis. |
Administration	It is administered parenterally and is therefore available in IV forms, which come in bags or bottles. It comes in several different concentrations, the most commonly used are **50 g/500 mL (10%)** and **100 g/500 mL (20%)**. Mannitol has the potential to crystallize – before administration it should be examined for crystals; if crystals are present, they can be dissolved by warming infusion fluid and gentle agitation. When using **mannitol 20% an in-line filter is recommended**.
Drug errors and safety	The osmotic effect of mannitol causes plasma volume expansion, which can precipitate heart failure. Prescribers should screen for heart failure prior to administration. Furthermore, due to its powerful diuretic effect patients can be at risk of **hypovolaemia** and **hypotension**. More importantly its administration can lead to electrolyte abnormalities such as **hypernatraemia** and **hypokalaemia**, which can precipitate **cardiac arrhythmias**. When considering repeat doses the clinician should be aware of the potential to cause high serum osmolarity and subsequent neurological effects.
Monitoring	The efficacy of mannitol is based on clinical signs or where available the results of monitoring such intracranial pressure monitoring. **Renal function, serum electrolytes, serum osmolality** and **urine osmolality** should be monitored.
Cost	Mannitol is a **cheap medicine**. The price depends on concentration: 500 mL of 10% mannitol is currently around £5, and 500 mL of 20% solution is currently £6–7.

Melatonin

CLINICAL PHARMACOLOGY

Why and when?	Melatonin is recommended for treatment of **sleep onset insomnia** and **delayed sleep phase syndrome**, when initiated under specialist supervision, although it is unlicensed. In adults it is also recommended short term for insomnia.
Absorption	Following oral administration, melatonin is poorly but **rapidly absorbed** from the gastrointestinal tract. Peak plasma concentrations are usually reached in **40 minutes**. Melatonin undergoes first-pass metabolism in the liver via cytochrome P450 enzymes where 90% is cleared and its systemic bioavailability is low. Recent studies in adult humans show an absolute bioavailability of only 3% but there is considerable inter-individual variability. It readily crosses the blood–brain barrier.
Biology	Melatonin (N-acetyl-5-methoxytryptamine) is synthesized in the **pineal gland** and helps to maintain the circadian rhythm with secretion high at night and low during the day. It acts on MT_1 and MT_2 G-protein coupled receptors found in the brain, retina and peripheral tissues. It is a **hypnotic** and results in drowsiness.
Clearance	Melatonin is metabolized by cytochrome P450 enzymes (particularly CYP1A2) in the liver. During this process, the melatonin metabolite 6-hydroxymelatonin is conjugated with sulfate and glucuronide and excreted via the kidneys; 2% of the melatonin administered is excreted unchanged. The half-life of melatonin is short and typically about **1–2 hours**. In order to extend the duration of action, melatonin is often given as a modified-release formulation. This results in slower absorption and a more sustained duration of action.

PRACTICAL PRESCRIBING

Dosing	For children the standard modified-release oral dose is 2–3 mg daily for 1–2 weeks. This is then increased, if necessary, to 4–6 mg daily, up to a maximum of 10 mg daily. Melatonin should be taken before bedtime.
Administration	**Melatonin is given orally at bedtime**. It is available as modified-release tablets or a specially prepared liquid formulation. The latter is a specially prepared medication and is very costly.
Drug errors and safety	Melatonin is very well tolerated even in high doses. Common side effects of melatonin include arthralgia, headaches, susceptibility to infection and abdominal, chest and musculoskeletal pain. Families need to be advised that melatonin can cause drowsiness and they should be warned against taking melatonin at any time other than just immediately preceding bedtime.
	As melatonin preparations contain lactose, it should not be taken by patients who have a lactose intolerance. Melatonin is present in breast milk and should be avoided if breastfeeding.
Monitoring	Patients should be initiated on melatonin by a specialist, and patients taking melatonin should be reviewed by a specialist every 6 months to ensure there is a continued requirement.
Cost	Melatonin is a **fairly expensive medication**. The cheapest formulation in the UK at the moment is Circadin® 2 mg modified-release tablets. A box of 30 2 mg tablets costs £15.39.

Meropenem

CLINICAL PHARMACOLOGY

Why and when?	Meropenem comes from the class of antibiotics called **carbapenems**. It is a relatively new antibiotic. Developed in the 1980s, it was first licensed for use in 1996. Most commonly it is used in severe infection, particularly when resistant organisms are suspected, i.e. in children with hospital-acquired infections or in those with poor response to initial treatment. It is used in many current treatment protocols for **febrile neutropenia**. It is sometimes used in the treatment of children and adults with more resistant *Pseudomonas aeruginosa* infections and cystic fibrosis (CF). It should be used sparingly, as **unnecessary use will promote the emergence of resistance**. It has a wide spectrum and is bactericidal against most Gram-negative and Gram-positive pathogenic bacteria.
Absorption	Meropenem **is given intravenously**. Following administration it distributes quickly and widely into tissues. It is given as an infusion over 15–30 minutes. It is minimally protein bound (2%). Meropenem provides adequate tissue concentration within 1 hour of receiving the dose.
Biology	Meropenem works by binding to the penicillin-binding proteins (PBPs) causing **cell lysis**. It is usually **bactericidal**. Its action is similar to related antibiotics including penicillins, cephalosporins and monobactams. However, it is **highly resistant to most β-lactamases**. Meropenem prevents bacteria from forming normal cell walls, which are essential for their survival. Meropenem covalently binds to PBPs (especially PBP2) intracellularly, which are involved in the biosynthesis of mucopeptides in bacterial cell walls. It is **bactericidal in most organisms** but bacteriostatic for *Listeria monocytogenes*. When resistance emerges, it is usually as a result of changes to the structure of PBPs.
Clearance	Meropenem has a **very short half-life**. It has a plasma half-life of approximately 1 hour in adults and children >2 years and 1.5–2 hours in infants and neonates. It is almost entirely excreted, unchanged by the kidneys. The clearance should be used as a guide for determining dosage for patients with renal impairment. Given the very short half-life some centres use **prolonged infusions**, which increase the amount of time that therapeutic serum levels are maintained.

PRACTICAL PRESCRIBING

Dosing	Dosing is dependent on the child's age, weight and the indication. After 7 days of age, doses are given 8-hourly. Higher doses are recommended in meningitis and severe infection. It is not licensed for use in children under 3 months of age.

Condition	Neonate up to 7 days	Neonate 7 days to 28 days	1 month–11 years (up to 50 kg)	1 month–11 years (over 50 kg)	12–17 years old
Aerobic/anaerobic Gram +VE/−VE Infections and hospital-acquired septicaemia	20 mg/kg every 12 h	20 mg/kg every 8 h	10–20 mg/kg every 8 h	0.5–1 g every 8 h	0.5–1 g every 8 h
Severe aerobic/ anaerobic Gram +VE/-VE Infections	40 mg/kg every 12 h	40 mg/kg every 8 h	–	–	–
Exacerbations of chronic lower respiratory tract infection in CF	–	–	40 mg/kg every 8 h	2 g every 8 h	2 g every 8 h
Meningitis	40 mg/kg every 12 h	40 mg/kg every 8 h	40 mg/kg every 8 h	2 g every 8 h	2 g every 8 h

Administration	Meropenem can be given as a slow IV injection (over 5 min) or as an infusion. Injections are only permissible for hospital-acquired septicaemia or severe infections. Given the relatively short half-life and the evidence suggesting benefits from prolonged infusion, when children are clinically stable **then infusions are probably preferable**. For IV infusion, dilute reconstituted solution further to a concentration of 1–20 mg/mL in 5% glucose or 0.9% sodium chloride solution and give over 15–30 min.
Drug errors and safety	Meropenem is related to penicillin and should be **avoided** if other antimicrobial options exist in children with **severe penicillin allergy**. However, the genuine **rates or cross-reactivity are low** and in clinical practice meropenem is often used, with caution, in children who report less severe penicillin reactions like rash or vomiting.
Monitoring	Monitor for immediate signs of hypersensitivity following administration.
Cost	Meropenem is **fairly expensive**. Currently a single vial of 500 mg powder for solution for injection costs between £8 and £10.

Methylphenidate (Ritalin®, Medikinet®, Concerta XL®, Equasym XL®)

CLINICAL PHARMACOLOGY

Why and when?	Methylphenidate, often better known by its trade name Ritalin®, is prescribed for **attention deficit hyperactivity disorder (ADHD)** in children aged 6 and over. The original forms of methylphenidate were immediate-release preparations. New modified-release preparations have been developed, which substantially alter the pharmacodynamics. These 'second-generation' products aim to deliver a rapid peak followed by sustained plasma concentrations. Rarely, it is also prescribed for narcolepsy in adults. In ADHD, it should be prescribed **after environmental modifications and other non-pharmacological approaches**. Treatment should be initiated under specialist supervision.
Absorption	Oral immediate-release methylphenidate is almost completely absorbed, but there is considerable variation in the speed of absorption between individuals. After a single oral dose of immediate-release methylphenidate **peak plasma levels are achieved within 1–3 hours** and the blood–brain barrier is rapidly crossed. It has a **bioavailability of approximately 20%**.
	Modified-release preparations consist of an immediate-release component of 22–50% of the total dose. **The modified-release forms are more slowly absorbed**. There are a range of innovative solutions that have been developed to delay release of methylphenidate including osmotic-controlled release oral delivery system (OROS®), Diffucaps® technology and SODAS® technology. OROS delivers the drug in a rigid tablet with a semipermeable outer membrane and one or more small laser-drilled holes within it. As water is absorbed through the semipermeable membrane osmotic pressure pushes active drug out of the tablet. Diffucaps and SODAS technology present drugs bound in microbeads within tablets with different coatings that variably release contents.
Biology	Methylphenidate is **a psychostimulant** and acts on the central nervous system as a **noradrenaline-dopamine reuptake inhibitor** (NDRI). Whilst it has an effect on both dopamine and noradrenaline transporters, methylphenidate is most active on dopamine transporters. This increases the amount of both dopamine and noradrenaline within the synaptic cleft, therefore increasing neurogenic transmission. This then increases **alertness, reduces fatigue and improves attention.**
Clearance	Once absorbed, methylphenidate is converted by the liver into ritalinic acid. It has a low binding to plasma proteins of 10–20%. The **plasma half-life of methylphenidate is 2–3 hours**. Ritalinic acid is mostly excreted in the urine within 2–4 days. A small amount is excreted in the faeces. A very small amount of methylphenidate is excreted in its unchanged form. The differences in serum levels over time achieved by different forms are attained by **delaying absorption of a proportion of the dose** in modified-release forms.

PRACTICAL PRESCRIBING

Dosing	Immediate-release preparations include Medikinet® and Ritalin. **These are given 2 or 3 times per day** usually at **4-hourly intervals**. In children over 5 a recommended starting dose is 5 mg 1–2 times a day. This is usually increased as necessary at weekly intervals by 5–10 mg per day (max dose 60 mg daily). It is often used 3 times a day at 4-hourly intervals. **Modified-release preparations are all given once daily**. The Concerta XL® formulation, which uses OROS delivery, has the lowest proportion of immediate-release methylphenidate (22%) and a higher starting dose of 18 mg is used. It can be increased at weekly intervals to 54 mg daily. The other forms, Equasym XL® with 30% immediate-release form and Medikinet XL® with 50% immediate-release form, start at 10 mg daily increasing at weekly intervals to maximum doses of 60 mg. Higher doses of all forms may be given under expert supervision.
Administration	Immediate-release oral preparations are available as tablets only. Modified-release preparations are available **as tablets or capsules**. The capsule form can be opened and contents sprinkled onto a tablespoon of apple sauce or yoghurt. If capsules are opened, then they should be **swallowed without chewing**. Equasym XL is best given before breakfast. Medikinet XL is best given with or after breakfast.
Drug errors and safety	Methylphenidate should only be started following a thorough biopsychosocial assessment. An electrocardiogram should be performed prior to initiation to **check for QT interval elongation**. If evidence of heart disease is found, or a family history of sudden cardiac death is reported, a cardiology opinion should be sought. Methylphenidate has a risk of psychological addiction. In high doses, it can lead to stimulant psychosis. Common side effects include gastrointestinal disturbance, **sleep disturbance**, a **reduction in appetite and growth retardation**. Sleep disturbance can be helped by altering medication times. Sudden withdrawal can lead to low mood and should be avoided.
Monitoring	Children should have their **height and weight monitored every 3–6 months** and this should be plotted on a growth chart to assess for weight loss. Pulse and blood pressure should be measured biannually and before and after changing doses. Patients should be advised to not abruptly stop taking this medication. It is typical to reduce and stop this medication during adolescence.
Cost	Many different preparations of methylphenidate are available. The immediate-release forms are cheapest with 30 × 10 mg tablets costing £5–6. Modified-release forms are more expensive at £24–32 for 30 tablets. **NHS spending on methylphenidate in the UK is currently £3–4m per month**.

Methotrexate

CLINICAL PHARMACOLOGY

Why and when?	Methotrexate is an **antimetabolite** with **antifolate activity**. It is used in **cancer treatment** and as a **steroid-sparing agent** in diseases that require **long-term immunosuppression.** At high doses, when used as chemotherapy, methotrexate inhibits synthesis of DNA, RNA and proteins. In lower doses it is **immunosuppressive** and inhibits chronic inflammatory pathways. It is used in a wide range of rheumatological, dermatological and gastroenterological conditions. Methotrexate is therefore a useful **steroid-sparing, disease-modifying drug** in autoimmune disorders.
Absorption	Data for absorption in humans are mostly based on adult studies. Oral bioavailability is **fairly good** at around 60% at doses of 30 mg/m^2. Higher doses begin to have lower bioavailability and there is some evidence in children that **subcutaneously administered methotrexate might be more effective**. The bioavailability following subcutaneous injection is close to 100%. The tolerability of oral and subcutaneous methotrexate is similar.
Biology	Methotrexate appears to exert its different effects through very different pathways. It **competitively inhibits dihydrofolate reductase** (DHFR). DHFR converts dihydrofolate into tetrahydrofolate, a methyl group shuttle required for the synthesis of purines, thymidylic acid and some amino acids. This prevents cell replication. The immunosuppressive effects are achieved at lower doses and work by inhibiting enzymes involved in purine metabolisms causing accumulation of adenosine. Methotrexate **also inhibits T-cell activation** by suppressing intercellular adhesion molecule expression. It also **increases T-cell apoptosis** and selectively **downregulates B-cells.**
Clearance	Intracellular and hepatic metabolism of methotrexate produces polyglutamates, which also inhibit DHFR and thymidylate synthetase. Methotrexate is also partially metabolized by intestinal flora, when taken orally. **Elimination is mainly by renal excretion** and depends on the dose and route of administration. The **half-life is quite variable**. Low doses delivered subcutaneously have a half-life of 2–3 hours. Higher doses, particularly those given orally, have half-lives of 10–15 hours. Despite this modest half-life, the **biological effects are sustained** and doses are **only given weekly**.

Prescribing tip — take great care in prescribing methotrexate and when preparing clinic and discharge letters. It is given weekly.

PRACTICAL PRESCRIBING

Dosing	The treatment dose for an acute flare and maintenance of remission in Crohn's disease is 15 mg/m^2 **weekly** (max 25 mg per dose), while treatment of disease activity (new or relapse) in autoimmune diseases such as lupus nephritis, scleroderma, juvenile dermatomyositis and juvenile idiopathic arthritis is within a dose range of 10–15 mg/m^2 **weekly**.
Administration	Methotrexate is available as tablets, liquid or subcutaneous injection. Common side effects include nausea and vomiting. **Folic acid is co-prescribed** to combat side effects and can be given up to 5 times a week, provided it **is not given on the same day as the methotrexate**. Co-administration of other antifolate drugs like **trimethoprim should be avoided**.
Drug errors and safety	Prescription errors are **common and potentially dangerous**. Great care must be taken when prescribing or re-prescribing methotrexate. Oral preparations are safe at room temperature, but **subcutaneous preparations need to be stored in a fridge**. Careful education of the family and child must occur before commencing methotrexate. It is only **given weekly** and long-term use results in **immunosuppression**. Clear instruction to omit doses of methotrexate while the child is either unwell with a fever or taking antibiotics for an infection should be given before the first dose is given. All patients must be screened for chickenpox, measles and tuberculosis (TB) infection or immunity before starting treatment.
Monitoring	Blood monitoring is required. When used in autoimmune disease, liver function and full blood counts should be taken after initiation **every 2 weeks for the first 6 weeks** and then **monthly for 3 months**. If the patient is stable then blood test must occur **at least every 3 months** whilst on treatment. Use in cancer will follow the cancer specific protocol. An increase of the liver enzymes (ALT and AST) by a factor of two is serious and requires omission of doses until normalization of blood results. The National Patient Safety Association recommend **monitoring diaries** and that written information about methotrexate is provided to families and patients starting methotrexate. Families should be warned **to report immediately** the onset of any feature **of blood disorders** (e.g. sore throat, bruising, mouth ulcers), **liver toxicity** (e.g. nausea, vomiting, abdominal discomfort, dark urine) and **respiratory effects** (e.g. shortness of breath).
Cost	Methotrexate **tablets are cheap**. 2.5 mg tablets can cost as little as 6p each. Oral solutions are more expensive: 2 mg/mL preparations cost between £95 and £125 for a 60–65 mL bottle. Pre-filled pens are available for subcutaneous injection. These vary in price but are typically £12–17 per dose.

Methylprednisolone

CLINICAL PHARMACOLOGY

Why and when?	Methylprednisolone is a **synthetic corticosteroid** used to **reduce inflammation and suppress the immune system**. It has a mainly glucocorticoid effect with some very limited mineralocorticoid effect. It can be given orally, intravenously, intramuscularly and by local injection. It is often given **intravenously as an infusion in very high doses** to regain control in autoimmune disease, e.g. **lupus**, **juvenile idiopathic arthritis** or **juvenile dermatomyositis**. High dose, short-burst therapy is often given for a few days and is referred to as 'pulsed' therapy. It was first described in the early 1970s as an effective treatment for **early graft rejection**.
Absorption	Methylprednisolone is **variably but rapidly absorbed from the gastrointestinal tract**. High oral doses are not used as they are likely to cause unacceptable gastrointestinal symptoms and so methylprednisolone in high doses is almost always used intravenously or as an injection directly into the affected area (e.g. a joint). When given intravenously, it reaches peak plasma concentrations **within minutes**. When given orally peak plasma concentrations are reached at 2–3 hours. Following administration it is rapidly distributed to the tissues.
Biology	The mode of action of corticosteroids is complex. Methylprednisolone has **significant glucocorticoid** and **modest mineralocorticoid effects**. It has relatively less mineralocorticoid effects than hydrocortisone or prednisolone, but more than dexamethasone (which has almost none).
	Endogenous cortisol is lipophilic. In the circulation, most cortisol is bound to corticosteroid-binding globulin (CBG) or albumin, and only a minority is free and biologically active. Acute stress leads to dramatic decreases in plasma CBG, increasing the activity. Other endogenous and exogenous steroids, including hydrocortisone, progesterone, prednisolone and aldosterone, compete for binding sites on CBG and high levels of one steroid will displace the others. In contrast, methylprednisolone **does not bind to CBG** and is therefore continuously biologically active.
	The aim of **pulse therapy** is to achieve a faster response and stronger efficacy and to **decrease the need for long-term use of systemic corticosteroids**. At very high doses steroids have somewhat different biological effects. These are not entirely understood. High doses dissolve in the cell membrane resulting in greater membrane stability and reduced cell function. Overall, pulses appear to downregulate activation of immune cells and reduce proinflammatory cytokine production.
Clearance	Methylprednisolone is metabolized in the liver to inactive glucuronide and sulfate metabolites. These inactive metabolites and small amounts of unchanged drug are excreted renally. The plasma half-life is around **3 hours** but the biological **half-life is fairly long at 18–36 hours.** There is evidence of diurnal variation in clearance, with a modest (20–25%) increase in clearance for doses given in the morning.

PRACTICAL PRESCRIBING

Dosing	Physiological (lower) doses of oral methylprednisolone are only infrequently used in children in the UK. Prednisolone or dexamethasone are more commonly used (see other chapters). When used the dose is 80% of the prednisolone dose. **Supraphysiological doses of methylprednisolone are given intravenously** as an infusion. Where available local guidelines and protocols should be followed. Typical doses for treatment of acute graft rejection are 10–20 mg/kg (up to a maximum of 1 g per day) for a maximum of 3 consecutive days. When given for severe erythema multiforme, lupus nephritis or systemic onset juvenile idiopathic arthritis the recommended dose is 10–30 mg/kg (up to a maximum of 1 g per day) either once daily or on alternate days for up to 3 doses.
Administration	There are many protocols for administration. Adverse effects are somewhat less common if infusions occur more slowly. The minimum infusion time is 30 minutes but most centres prefer **minimum infusion times to be 1 hour**. Slower infusion rates reduce the incidence of anaphylaxis, hypertension and hyperglycaemia. Methylprednisolone should be diluted with 0.9% sodium chloride solution to make a total volume of 100 mL. Prior to and during infusion it is necessary to monitor the **heart rate**, respiratory rate, **blood pressure and temperature**. Urine should be checked for glucose each morning. Children may require glucose monitoring, particularly if they have diabetes.
Monitoring	**Growth parameters must be monitored**. Children receiving pulsed methylprednisolone commonly need inflammatory markers and other blood tests (full blood count, liver function tests, creatine kinase) to monitor their underlying disease.
Side effects	Side effects **are common**. During administration facial flushing, a metallic taste in the mouth, hyperactivity, **mood changes**, blurred vision and lethargy are all common. If stinging occurs during infusion, then slowing the rate or giving as a more dilute solution can help. When used in short bursts, adrenal suppression is uncommon. However, increased appetite, abnormal behaviour (aggression), hypertension and impaired diabetic control are all commonly encountered. Psychiatric reactions are seen (including euphoria, insomnia, irritability, mood lability, suicidal thoughts and behavioural disturbances) and families should be warned of these and the risk of severe infection with chickenpox and measles if significant immunosuppression is anticipated.
Cost	Methylprednisolone is **fairly cheap**. Intravenous Solu-Medrone™ costs £17.30/g. Oral preparations are available in tablets of 2 mg, 4 mg, 16 mg and 100 mg at a cost from £3.88 to £48.32. Depo-Medrone® suspension, usually used intra-articularly comes in 40 mg, 80 mg and 120 mg vials (same concentration) at a cost of £3.44 to £8.96 per vial.

Metronidazole

CLINICAL PHARMACOLOGY

Why and when?	Metronidazole is an **antibiotic.** Its activity is limited to **anaerobic** bacteria and protozoa. Anaerobic bacteria are present in the normal flora of the oropharynx, gastrointestinal tract and genital tracts. Metronidazole is therefore used to treat infections originating from these systems and is often combined with antibiotics targeting aerobic organisms. The most common use in paediatrics is in the treatment of **gastrointestinal infections**, which includes necrotizing enterocolitis or pseudomembranous colitis secondary to *Clostridium difficile*. **Dental infections** and **pelvic inflammatory disease** can also be treated with metronidazole. Anaerobic protozoan infections occur less commonly but include amoebiasis, giardiasis and trichomoniasis. Metronidazole is used as a component of *Helicobacter pylori* eradication therapy or to aid healing in fistulating Crohn's disease.
Absorption and distribution	Metronidazole is **well absorbed orally** with a bioavailability of 98.9%. Despite its poor protein binding capacity, metronidazole is **widely distributed** throughout fluid compartments (including cerebrospinal fluid) and reaches a peak plasma concentration at 2–3 hours following oral administration. There is bioequivalence between oral and intravenous (IV) routes with the latter being reserved for neonates and severe infections. Metronidazole is available as a rectal preparation, which is well absorbed and can be considered as an alternative if required. Metronidazole achieves high concentrations in breast milk and may cause a bitter taste.
Biology	Metronidazole is a synthetic nitroimidazole antimicrobial, which is **bactericidal**. It passively diffuses into susceptible organisms and is converted to its active form by reduction of the nitro group. This metabolic pathway is only present in anaerobic organisms as the presence of oxygen inhibits the reduction process. The result is a cytotoxic molecule that interferes with energy metabolism and **inhibits nucleic acid synthesis** leading to cell death.
Clearance	Metronidazole is hydroxylated and conjugated by cytochrome P450 in the liver and excreted in the urine. Both the original compound and metabolites show *in vitro* activity against anaerobic organisms. The **half-life is 8 hours** with the metabolism in children older than 4 years being similar to adults. Neonates have a reduced ability to eliminate metronidazole and the half-life is thought to be inversely related to birth weight and gestational age. For this reason the dosing interval is extended in preterm infants.

PRACTICAL PRESCRIBING

Dosing	The dose and frequency of administration depends on the type of infection and the age of the child. For anaerobic bacterial infections the usual dose is **7.5 mg/kg (maximum 400 mg)** for both IV and oral preparations. For children 2 months of age and older this is administered 3 times per day. For IV administration, loading doses are recommended in neonates and infants up to 2 months of age at 15 mg/kg. Subsequent doses are 7.5 mg/kg at differing intervals dependent on the corrected gestational age. The doses required to treat protozoal infection are higher and often for a shorter duration. Doses are reduced to one-third of the recommended dose and administered once daily in severe liver disease. No dose change is recommended in renal disease but the patient must be monitored for adverse effects.
Administration	Metronidazole is available in various preparations. Oral formulations can be obtained as both tablets (200 mg, 400 mg and 500 mg) and suspension (200 mg/5 mL). IV metronidazole is available in 500 mg/ 100 mL and should be administered as an infusion over 20–30 minutes. Metronidazole can also be administered via a suppository for systemic use or topically in the form of a gel or cream for specific indications.
Side effects and interactions	Metronidazole **inhibits cytochrome P450** and can interact with other medicines metabolized by this group of enzymes. When metronidazole is administered alongside one of these drugs, their serum levels can rise above the therapeutic range and cause adverse effects. If metronidazole is given alongside a medication known to induce cytochrome P450 then its antimicrobial effect will be less due to enhanced metabolism leading to reduced plasma concentrations.
	Metronidazole **can cause a metallic taste** and non-specific gastro-intestinal disturbance. In treatment courses involving a high dose or long duration there is an increased risk of peripheral neuropathy and caution should be used with the use of other medication causing peripheral neuropathy.
Monitoring	Monitoring of metronidazole plasma concentration is not recommended routinely; however, in treatment courses lasting **longer than 10 days** it is advisable to consider performing a **full blood count** and **liver function test** due to the adverse effects associated with long-term therapy.
Cost	The cost of metronidazole varies, dependent on the preparation. 200 mg **tablets are cheap** with a 7-day course costing £1.70. The oral suspension is more expensive, costing £32.93 for 100 mL. The IV infusion costs £3.19 per 500 mg/100 mL bag.

Midazolam

CLINICAL PHARMACOLOGY

Why and when?	Midazolam is a short-acting benzodiazepine with rapid onset of action. It has **anticonvulsant**, **anxiolytic, amnesic** and **muscle relaxant** activity. The amnesic, sedative and anticonvulsant properties are brought about by γ-aminobutyric acid (GABA) accumulation and occupation of benzodiazepine receptors. Anxiolytic properties are related to increasing the concentration glycine inhibitory neurotransmitter. Recent evidence indicates that **midazolam may be as effective as lorazepam in curtailing seizures** during status epilepticus (SE).
Absorption	The absolute bioavailability of midazolam **depends significantly upon the route of administration**. Whilst there is inter-individual variability approximately 25% of an oral dose and 18% of a rectal dose are absorbed. It is fairly efficiently absorbed through the oral or nasal mucosa and approximately 50% of an oromucosal (buccal) or nasal dose is absorbed. The peak effect is seen almost immediately with intravenous (IV) dosing, within 15 minutes for intramuscular (IM) dosing at 30 min for rectal or buccal midazolam and about 1 hour for oral midazolam. Midazolam is highly bound to plasma protein.
Biology	Midazolam's mechanism of action **is similar to lorazepam and other benzodiazepines**, in that it acts primarily through potentiating the benzodiazepine–GABA$_A$ receptor complex. This enhances the inhibitory action of γ-aminobutyric acid type A (GABA$_A$) by increasing the number of chloride channel openings resulting in the hyperpolarization of neurons. SE is thought to result from a failure of the normal mechanisms for seizure termination, in particular, a decrease in GABA$_A$ receptor function and an increase in glutamate receptor density.
Clearance	The half-life of midazolam is between 1.5 and 2.5 hours, which is **about 20-fold shorter than that of diazepam**. It is mainly eliminated by hydroxylation to form 1-hydroxymidazolam by CYP3A4 and CYP3A5 enzymes. 1-Hydroxymidazolam **has a significant sedative effect**. Finally, this metabolite undergoes glucuronidation before excretion into urine. Hepatic CYP3A4 activity appears in the liver during the first weeks of life; it is thus lower in neonate than adult liver, resulting in **reduced midazolam clearance in neonates**. CYP3A4 and CYP3A5 activities reach adult levels between 3 and 12 months of postnatal age.
Route of administration and clinical effects	The **route of administration** affects the pharmacokinetics and, to an extent, **influences the clinical effects** exerted by midazolam and its metabolites. IV or mucosal (nasal or buccal routes) forms avoid hepatic first-pass metabolism. Oral midazolam reaches a slower and lower peak plasma concentration than that achieved by IV or mucosal administration, therefore it has somewhat less amnesic and anxiolytic qualities.

PRACTICAL PRESCRIBING

Dosing	For the treatment of seizures, midazolam is usually given **by the oromucosal (buccal) route**. The doses are: <3 months: 300 micrograms (mcg)/kg; 3–11 months: 2.5 mg; 1–4 years: 5 mg; 5–9 years: 7.5 mg; and >9 years: 10 mg. Doses may be repeated at 10 min intervals. If using the IV route then an initial dose of 150–200 mcg/kg is followed by a continuous IV infusion of 60 mcg/kg/h, which is increased in steps of 60 mcg/kg/h every 15 min (max. dose 300 mcg/kg/h) until seizures are controlled.
	Midazolam can be used as sedation for procedures, for children receiving intensive care and as a premedication. It is also sometimes used in the palliative care setting both for uncontrolled seizures and agitation. Doses vary considerably but it should only be used by those familiar with its use and with training in its use.
Side effects and considerations for use	General side effects of all benzodiazepines include **amnesia**, confusion, **drowsiness**, hypotension, dizziness, restlessness and paradoxical aggression/excitement. Skin rashes, anaphylaxis, bronchospasm, involuntary movements, urinary retention and convulsions (more common in neonates) can occur. Midazolam commonly causes a decrease in conscious level. This may be accompanied by **respiratory depression and vomiting**. Care needs to be taken particularly when used outside hospital. Parents and carers are advised to call an ambulance for support the first time that they administer a dose in the home or school setting. Parents should receive appropriate training in use and resuscitation before prescribing. A helpful information leaflet for parents is available at https://www.medicinesforchildren.org.uk/midazolam-stopping-seizures.
	There have been reports of over dosage when high-strength midazolam has been used for conscious sedation. The use of high-strength midazolam (5 mg/mL in 2 mL and 10 mL ampoules or 2 mg/mL in 5 mL ampoules) should be restricted to general anaesthesia, intensive care, palliative care, or other situations where the risk has been assessed. It is advised that the **antidote** and selective GABA$_A$ antagonist **flumazenil** is available when midazolam is used, to reverse the effects if necessary. When used as infusions for prolonged periods it accumulates in tissues and its effects may be prolonged and withdrawal reactions are common. However, there is no need to monitor midazolam levels in clinical practice.
Cost	IV preparations of midazolam **are inexpensive** and cost between 5p and 20p per milligram depending upon the solution strength. It is available as solutions of 2 mg/2 mL, 5 mg/5 mL and 10 mg/2 mL for injection. **Oromucosal** forms in pre-filled syringes are **significantly more costly**. The cost of a single oromucosal pre-filled syringe is between £20 and £25. These can be prescribed for parents of children with known seizures to keep as an emergency treatment for seizures out of hospital.

Montelukast

CLINICAL PHARMACOLOGY

Why and when?

Montelukast is a relatively new medication, introduced in the late 1990s, for the **treatment of asthma**. In the UK it most commonly prescribed in children who are not optimally managed on a combination of salbutamol and inhaled corticosteroids (ICS). While the evidence for this is not conclusive, there does appear to be some benefit in terms of lung function and frequency of asthma attacks when compared with salbutamol and ICS alone. It is also used to treat younger children (<5 years) with **recurrent viral induced wheeze**. However, whilst some centres advocate a trial period of 6–8 weeks followed by a review of symptoms, the evidence for this approach is limited. It has also shown some benefit in the treatment of **seasonal rhinitis**. It is licensed in the UK for the treatment of seasonal rhinitis in adolescents >15 years old. The clinical efficacy of montelukast appears to vary significantly between different individuals with a clinical response rate of between 25% and 60%, which may be caused by genetic variability in its metabolism. In all children, clinical response (or lack of it) should be carefully documented. **If it is ineffective, then it should be discontinued**. The main advantage of montelukast is that it is usually easer to administer than inhaled medications.

Absorption

Montelukast is **well absorbed** from the small intestine following oral administration with a somewhat greater bioavailability in patients who are fasting (73% for 5 mg tablet) when compared to fed individuals (63%). It demonstrates **rapid absorption** following oral administration and the time to peak blood concentration is around 2 hours for a 4 mg tablet or 2–5 hours for a 5 mg tablet. In adults montelukast demonstrates a volume of distribution of between 8 and 11 litres with >99% plasma protein binding.

Biology

Montelukast belongs to a class of medications termed selective **leukotriene receptor antagonists** (LTRA). It **inhibits the cysteinyl leukotriene receptor** (CysLT1). Cysteinyl leukotrienes are released from cells such as eosinophils and mast cells and mediate a pro-inflammatory process. In the airways, this contributes to the typical triad of mucosal oedema, increased secretions and smooth muscle contraction/proliferation, which contribute to the pathophysiology of asthma. Montelukast exerts its clinical benefits by **inhibiting the release of leukotrienes** and thus dampening this inflammatory cascade.

Clearance

Montelukast is **extensively metabolized in the liver** via the enzymes: CYP3A4, 2C8 and 2C9 and is **excreted almost exclusively in bile** (86%) with less than 0.2% excreted via the urine. In children between 6 and 23 months of age, systemic exposure to montelukast is greater than in adults (at equivalent dose) due to reduced hepatic metabolism of the immature liver. The elimination half-life for healthy adults is between 2.7 and 5.5 hours. It is usually given once daily to children with asthma.

PRACTICAL PRESCRIBING

Dosing	Montelukast is licensed for use in children >6 months of age for the **treatment of asthma**. Between the ages of 6 months and 5 years, 4 mg should be taken once daily in the evening. In those aged 6–14 years this dose increases to 5 mg and in those between 15 and 17 years, a dose of 10 mg is advised. The dose is the same for the treatment of seasonal rhinitis although it is only licensed for children >14 years for this indication.
Administration	Montelukast is only available in **oral preparations**. At lower doses (4–5 mg), it can be administered as either a chewable tablet or granules; however, the stronger preparation (10 mg) is only available in the as a tablet. Unusually, both the chewable tablet and granule forms actually taste quite nice. Palatability is not a common issue.

Dosing for **asthma is recommended in the evening**; however, patients with allergic rhinitis may take montelukast in the morning or evening depending on their individual preference. The chewable tablet may be administered with or without food but granules should be administered directly into the mouth, dissolved in 5 mL of cool milk formula/breast milk or mixed with a spoonful of soft food, such as yoghurt or vegetable/fruit puree. The granules should not be added to liquid and must be administered within 15 minutes of opening the packet. |
Drug errors and safety	Montelukast should be considered a relatively safe medication with few serious adverse events. As it is almost exclusively metabolized by the liver, caution should be taken when administering to those with hepatic impairment to avoid excessive drug accumulation. Common adverse events in children include abdominal pain, headache, **hyperkinesia** and **increased thirst** (which is often transient if treatment is continued). Less commonly children may report **abnormal dreams** (and night terrors) or **behavioural changes** following administration. In some instances this may be a reason for discontinuing treatment. These symptoms appear to improve once medication is discontinued. Very rarely, Churg–Strauss syndrome has been reported.
Monitoring	Efficacy of montelukast should be monitored by observing asthma symptoms, peak flow and other lung function tests. **Children should be monitored for behavioural changes such as low mood and suicidal thoughts**. Montelukast should be discontinued if it is ineffective or if children develop a vasculitic rash, eosinophilia or worsening pulmonary symptoms.
Cost	Montelukast is **more expensive and less effective** than most brands of low-dose ICS for treatment of asthma. In the UK, a pack of 28 chewable montelukast tablets costs £25.69. Granules are slightly cheaper at £24.41 for 28 sachets.

Morphine

CLINICAL PHARMACOLOGY

Why and when?	Morphine is a **potent opioid analgesic** with a quick onset of action. It is used primarily as **analgesia** for **moderate-to-severe pain**; however, it can also cause sedative, hypnotic and anti-peristaltic effects. Morphine is also used in **neonatal opioid withdrawal**, and a **sedative for premedication** in neonates and infants for intubation and ventilation.
Absorption and distribution	Morphine is usually administered orally to children. It can be given as immediate-release or in sustained-release forms. The onset of action of immediate-release oral morphine solution usually occurs within 15–30 minutes of administration and peaks at 1 hour. It rapidly and **readily crosses the blood–brain barrier**. When given orally, doses have to be up to 5–6 times higher than IV doses. This is due in part to a **significant first-pass metabolism**. The relative bioavailability of oral morphine is c.20–25% in healthy adults. Morphine has a low affinity to plasma protein of around 35%.
	Sustained-release morphine preparations (MST Continus®, Morphgesic®SR, Zomorph, Filnarine®SR and MXL®) achieve peak plasma concentrations more slowly (c.2.5 hours in adults and longer in many children). These may take up to 12 hours to achieve maximum effects in children and in the initiation phase may need to be co-administered with immediate-release preparations or other analgesics.
Biology	Morphine binds to μ **opioid receptors.** These are predominantly located in the dorsal horn of the spinal cord, cerebral cortex and gastrointestinal tract. These receptors are involved with the **transmission of pain** signals around the central nervous system, respiratory control and gut motility. When morphine binds to these receptors there are several clinical effects. Morphine results in **analgesia**, **sedation**, **hypotension**, **euphoria**, **reduced respiration** and **reduced bowel motility**. Morphine has an important active metabolite called morphine-6-glucoronide; this accounts for 85% of the effects that are given when morphine is taken. μ (mu) and κ (kappa) opioid receptors are also located in the nucleus accumbens, which is where sensation, euphoria and reward are triggered. Continuous use leads to rapid tachyphylaxis and dependency.
Clearance	The biological half-life of immediate-release morphine and its metabolites is **2–3 hours** in infants and older children. It is significantly longer in preterm infants (c.9 hours) and term neonates up to 2 months (c.6.5 hours). Most morphine is eliminated following **glucuronidation**. A small proportion (2–10%) of morphine and most of its metabolites are eliminated via the urine. Hepatic and renal impairment will reduce the clearance.

PRACTICAL PRESCRIBING

Dosing	For the treatment of pain, morphine is usually given orally. Starting doses are age- and weight-dependent. It is usually given every 6 hours in children <6 months, 4-hourly in older children.

Typical starting doses are: <3 months: 50–100 micrograms (mcg)/kg; 3 month–2 years: 100–200 mcg/kg; 2–11 years: 200–300 mcg/kg max. dose 10 mg; 12–17 years: 2.5–10 mg. All doses must be checked against local protocols and **adjusted according to clinical response** and some children will need more to achieve adequate analgesia.

For chronic pain, modified-release tablets can be given; this can be dosed in the same way as oral morphine. For IV doses of morphine a lower dose is needed due to missing first pass metabolism. Typical doses for children receiving infusions are 10–40 mcg/kg/h. |
| Side effects and considerations for use | General side effects of all opioids include confusion, constipation, drowsiness, dry mouth, euphoria, hallucinations, headache, nausea, palpitations, skin reactions and urinary retention. It causes pupillary constriction. Morphine can also result in an **anaphylactoid reaction**, a result of a direct action on mast cells. Care must be given when morphine is first administered as nausea, vomiting and respiratory depression are common. Constipation is so common with prolonged use that it may be helpful to co-prescribe a laxative. After prolonged use (or exposure) then withdrawal is common. The features of withdrawal are the opposite to the clinical effects of morphine. Children who are withdrawing have diarrhoea, dilated pupils, sweat, are anxious, breathless and in pain. Some may have seizures. Morphine readily crosses the placenta and babies born to mothers taking morphine in any form may suffer withdrawal. This is called neonatal abstinence syndrome.

In overdose then, a specific short-acting antidote, **naloxone**, is useful. Naloxone is a competitive agonist for the μ opioid receptor along with other receptors and is effective at reversing an overdose but due to its short half-life after initiation further doses or infusion will be required.

Morphine solution at lower concentrations is not a controlled drug (i.e. 10 mg/5 mL); higher concentrations (i.e. >13 mg/5 mL) and tablets are controlled. |
| Cost | Morphine is **cheap in all forms**. IV preparations cost around £1–5 depending on the dose and if it is infused or directly injected. Oral morphine is the cheapest form of morphine, which is currently around 8p–9p for 10 mg of oral morphine solution (Oramorph) in the UK. Modified-release morphine is only slightly more expensive, costing around 6p–7p for 10 mg of MST Continus but up to £1.50 per dose for 200 mg of the once-daily MXL preparation. |

Macrogols

CLINICAL PHARMACOLOGY

Why and when?	Macrogols are commonly used laxatives. They are now often used as **first-line medical treatment for constipation** when lifestyle and dietary changes have been ineffective. They can be given either as a part of a disimpaction regimen or as part of a maintenance regimen for those with chronic constipation. They are available in paediatric preparations, which contain half the macrogol '3350' and electrolyte loads of adult preparations. Preparations also contain potassium chloride, sodium bicarbonate and sodium chloride and must be taken with an **adequate volume of water**. They come in a variety of different flavours ranging from plain, to lemon and lime, to chocolate.
Absorption	The macrogol '3350' component of the varying preparations is **not absorbed**. The electrolytes that form part of the preparations are aimed at maintaining rather than altering serum electrolytes.
Biology	In adults the large intestine typically receives about 8 L of liquid faeces per day. Normally the large bowel reabsorbs nearly all the fluid resulting in 250–300 g of faeces being eliminated. Macrogol '3350' is an inert polymer of ethylene glycol, which acts as an **osmotic laxative**. This opposes water reabsorption within the lumen of the large bowel. This increases the water content and volume of stool. The increase in stool bulk also helps to improve overall gut function and motility and over time less is needed to have a similar effect. As correctly prepared macrogol '3350' is taken with fluid it reduces the dehydrating effect associated with some osmotic laxatives.
Clearance	Macrogol '3350' is virtually unabsorbed from the gastrointestinal tract and is **excreted, unaltered, in faeces**. Any macrogol '3350' that enters the systemic circulation is excreted in urine.
Dosing	Children presenting with faecal impaction will initially need higher doses to provide relief. Once the child is opening their bowels regularly, the dose can be reduced. The dose is typically adjusted to ensure that the stool is soft and sausage shaped. If a child is passing liquid stool, they may need careful assessment. If there are still significant palpable stools in the abdomen then liquid stool may reflect **overflow diarrhoea** and a further disimpaction regimen may be required. The required doses are variable between children and influenced by other factors such as diet.

PRACTICAL PRESCRIBING

| Dosing (continued) | **For faecal impaction*** (typical recommended number of sachets of macrogol '3350') : |

	Day 1	Day 2	Day 3	Day 4	Day 5	Day 6	Day 7
1–5 years	2	4	4	6	6	8	8
6–11 years	4	6	8	10	12	12	12
12+ years	4	6	8	8	8	8	8

*Children under 12 should receive a paediatric preparation.

For treatment of chronic constipation (typical maintenance phase doses):
Children under 1 year: 0.5–1 sachet per day.
Children 1–2 years: 1 sachet per day (max. 4 per day).
Children 2–5 years: 1 sachet per day (max. 4 per day).
Children 6–11 years: 2 sachets per day (max. 4 per day).
Children >12 years: 1–2 sachets of **adult macrogol** '3350' preparation.

| Administration | Macrogol '3350' preparations are available as a liquid and powdered preparation. However, paediatric preparations (half strength) are only available as a powdered preparation and as either plain (no added colours, flavours or sweeteners) or chocolate flavour. Half-strength sachets should be dissolved in 62.5 mL of water. Full strength needs to be dissolved in at least 125 mL of water. **This is vital in ensuring the medicine works** and also minimizes the risk of dehydration. It is not necessary for the child to drink all of the sachets in one sitting, after making it **should be kept in the refrigerator**. It may be spaced throughout the day (12 h) and can be given with squash, smoothies or frozen into ice lollies; straws are also useful if palatability is a problem. Movicol® liquid can be taken as directed and does not need to be diluted in water. |

| Drug errors and safety | All macrogol '3350' preparations can **contribute to dehydration**. If the child is feeling sick or is vomiting, the advice is to continue to give treatment less frequently whilst ensuring that the child receives adequate oral fluid hydration. Preparations also contain potassium chloride at a concentration of 5.4 mmol/L (when reconstituted correctly). Care should be taken for those with renal or cardiovascular impairment. At very high doses it can cause impaired consciousness, impaired gag reflex and reflux oesophagitis. It is advised that no more than 4 paediatric sachets or 2 adult sachets are given within 1 hour. Monitoring of levels is not required but doses should be adjusted according to stool consistency. |

| Cost | Movicol is a relatively inexpensive medicine. Movicol Paediatric Plain/Chocolate costs £4.38 for 30 sachets. CosmoCol® Paediatric oral powder and Laxido® Paediatric Plain are slightly cheaper at c.£3. |

Omalizumab

CLINICAL PHARMACOLOGY

Why and when?	Omalizumab is a monoclonal antibody that specifically binds to free immunoglobulin E (IgE). It is a **biological** agent. It is used as an add-on therapy in the treatment of **severe persistent allergic asthma** and to treat chronic spontaneous urticaria in older children who have had a poor response to conventional treatment including antihistamines. It is administered as a subcutaneous injection.
Absorption	Omalizumab is administered subcutaneously every 2 to 4 weeks. The precise regimen is based on serum IgE concentration and body weight (see Appendix 2). Omalizumab is absorbed with an average absolute **bioavailability of 62%**. After injection, **omalizumab is absorbed slowly**, reaching peak serum concentrations after an average of 6–8 days.
Biology	Immediate (Type I) hypersensitivity reactions are **IgE mediated**. IgE plays a central role in the development of **atopy**. In atopic (allergic) individuals, exposure to an allergen initiates a series of events that leads to the production of allergen specific IgE (sIgE). Subsequent antigen exposure allows binding and cross-linking of sIgE on mast cells, basophils and eosinophils, leading to cytokine and histamine release. Omalizumab is a **recombinant humanized IgG1 monoclonal antibody** that **inhibits the binding of IgE to the high affinity receptor** FcER1 on the surface of mast cells and basophils. This anti-IgE antibody forms complexes with free IgE.
Clearance	Clearance of omalizumab **is complex**. The **liver reticuloendothelial system** and **endothelial cells** are responsible for the elimination of IgG and omalizumab : IgE complexes. The degradation products are recycled to smaller peptides and amino acids, which can be utilized in protein synthesis. Clinical studies have also found that small amounts of intact IgG are also excreted in bile.

Whilst the **elimination of omalizumab : IgE is dose dependent**, there will be rapid complex formation with any serum IgE once omalizumab enters the blood. The aim of therapy is to temporarily suppress IgE responses by binding and inactivating IgE non-specifically. As doses are titrated to total IgE levels, then free serum levels are relatively low but constant. In general, omalizumab : IgE serum elimination half-life is around 25 days and doses need to be repeated every 2–4 weeks depending upon the serum IgE levels and weight of the child. |

PRACTICAL PRESCRIBING

Dosing	The appropriate dose and frequency of omalizumab for children with **severe persistent allergic asthma** are determined by baseline IgE (IU/mL) and body weight (kg) measured **before the start of treatment** (see Appendix 2). Omalizumab is a very expensive treatment and should only be initiated by centres with expertise in treating severe asthma. Children with very high serum IgE levels (>1500 IU/mL) or who are very heavy with moderately high serum IgE are not suitable for treatment with omalizumab. For older children (12–17 years) and adults with **severe persistent chronic spontaneous urticaria** who have had an inadequate response to other oral treatments the dose is **300 mg every 4 weeks**.
Administration	Omalizumab is administered via pre-filled subcutaneous injection in 75 mg and 150 mg solutions. The syringes should be stored in a refrigerator and protected from light. **The syringe should be taken out 20 minutes before to reach room temperature**. Manufacturers recommend that the injection is given in the arm or thigh. Most children dislike these injections and play therapists and experienced nurse specialists are invaluable in reducing the psychological burden of this treatment.
Drug errors and safety	Omalizumab is to be used with caution in autoimmune diseases. Any reduction in serum IgE increases the susceptibility to parasitic infections. Common side effects include fever, gastrointestinal discomfort, headache and skin reactions. Eosinophilic granulomatosis with polyangiitis (Churg–Strauss syndrome) occurs rarely. Severe hypersensitivity reactions (**anaphylaxis**) can also occur following treatment, immediately or sometimes >24 hours after the injection.
Monitoring	**At 16 weeks** after commencing omalizumab therapy patients should be reassessed by their specialist asthma or allergy physician **for treatment effectiveness** before continuation.
Cost	Omalizumab is **very expensive**. It costs £256.15 for a single 150 mg pre-filled syringe. Annual costs for a child with severe asthma at the highest dose range are more than £16,000 for drugs alone.

Omeprazole

CLINICAL PHARMACOLOGY

Why and when?	Omeprazole is a **proton pump inhibitor** (PPI) that reduces the acidity of gastric secretions. It can be used during the neonatal period and into adulthood. In the paediatric population it is mainly used to treat **gastro-oesophageal reflux disease** (GORD), especially that associated with mucosal damage. It is also used as part of triple therapy against *Helicobacter pylori* infection and in the treatment of gastric and duodenal ulcers. It has a role in **protection of the gastric mucosa** when a child or young person has to take a prolonged course of non-steroidal anti-inflammatory drugs (NSAIDs) or steroids. It is useful in Zollinger–Ellison syndrome (including cases resistant to other forms of treatment). For children with cystic fibrosis it **enhances the activity of pancreatic enzyme supplements**, which require an alkaline environment for optimal effectiveness.
Absorption	Omeprazole is **rapidly and readily absorbed** from the gastrointestinal tract. It has a bioavailability of approximately 60%. Peak plasma concentrations are reached within half an hour. Those in protective coatings can take longer, up to 3 hours. The time for mucosal healing and relief of symptoms to occur is, however, much slower at around 2 weeks plus. The clinical effects of omeprazole (and other PPIs) are **not dependent upon plasma levels**, but rather they appear to depend upon the level **within the parietal cells of the gastric mucosa**. Omeprazole is a weak base, and thus accumulates within the acidic space adjacent to parietal cells in the stomach.
Biology	PPIs are prodrugs, which **need to be activated by acid**. Omeprazole works by **blocking the action of** the hydrogen–potassium adenosine triphosphatase enzyme ($H^+/K^+-ATPase$) system of the gastric parietal cells. It accumulates in the acid secretory canaliculus of the parietal cells. There it converts to its reactive form, a cation that covalently binds to the $H^+/K^+-ATPase$ enzyme. This ultimately disrupts hydrogen ion transport and significantly reduces gastric acid secretion.
Clearance	Omeprazole reaching the plasma is **rapidly metabolized by the liver**, a process dependent on the cytochrome P450 system. It has a half-life of less than 1 hour and is usually completely eliminated from the plasma within 3–4 hours. This is in contrast to its extended anti-acid action *in vivo*. The two major plasma metabolites are sulfone and hydroxyomeprazole, neither of which contributes to its antisecretory activity. Around 80% of a given dose is excreted in the urine.

PRACTICAL PRESCRIBING

Dosing	For all indications except eradication of *Helicobacter pylori* the recommended oral doses are 700 micrograms (mcg)/kg for children <2 years of age with maximum doses of 1.4 mg/kg–3 mg/kg depending upon age and gestation. For older children the oral dose depends upon age and weight. For 10–19 kg children 10 mg once daily is initially used (max dose 20 mg). For those over 20 kg a dose of 20 mg once daily is used and can be increased to a maximum of 40 mg daily.
	For eradication of *Helicobacter pylori*, the recommended oral dose is 1–2 mg/kg (max. dose 40 mg) in children >1 year.
Administration	Omeprazole comes in capsule, tablet, liquid and dispersible forms. Some capsule forms (i.e. Losec MUPS®) can be opened and mixed with fruit juice or yoghurt. Liquid omeprazole is very expensive and so rarely prescribed and has been supplanted in many instances by esomeprazole. If giving via an enteral feeding tube, Losec MUPS or the contents of a capsule must be dispersed in a large volume of water or it tends to **precipitate and block the tube**. It is most commonly a **once-a-day medication** taken in the mornings.
Drug errors and safety	Side effects include abdominal pain, altered bowel habit, nausea, vomiting, dry mouth and dizziness, headache or altered sensations and mood. Less common but serious effects are leukopenia, thrombocytopenia, visual disturbances, alopecia, renal disturbance and gynaecomastia. Whilst PPIs are widely used, long-term administration **increases risk of gastrointestinal infections** including *Clostridium difficile* and the risk of **osteoporosis**. Observational studies have suggested that PPIs may increase the risk of **pneumonia** but the mechanism and strength of association in children are unclear.
Monitoring	Omeprazole can precipitate or worsen hypomagnesaemia. Consider checking serum magnesium concentrations before and during prolonged treatment, especially when used with other drugs that cause hypomagnesaemia such as **diuretics** or **digoxin**.
Cost	Whilst some forms of omeprazole are cheap, the **prices for omeprazole vary dramatically** between manufacturer and form of drug. Typical costs for a month supply of 10 mg daily can be as low as £1.34 for capsules, £8.40 for Losec MUPS and £137.24 for liquid formulations. It is important to stipulate the type of omeprazole required for a child if it is not the cheapest available form.

Ondansetron

CLINICAL PHARMACOLOGY

Why and when?	Ondansetron is an **antiemetic** that is used for treatment of nausea and vomiting. It is currently licensed in children for the prevention and treatment of nausea and vomiting postoperatively and with chemotherapy- and radiotherapy-induced symptoms. Whilst there is evidence that it may be beneficial in children with **acute gastroenteritis**, this is not a licensed indication. However, individual trusts may have separate guidance for off-label use of ondansetron in acute gastroenteritis.
Absorption	Orally administered ondansetron is completely absorbed within the gastrointestinal tract, both passively and actively. However, it is subjected to extensive first-pass metabolism within the liver meaning the **actual bioavailability is around 60%** of the administered dose. Peak serum concentrations are reached within 90 minutes of administration. When given intravenously, peak serum concentration is reached within 10 minutes of administration.
Biology	Ondansetron is a first-generation 5-hydroxytryptamine (5-HT$_3$) receptor-antagonist. The mechanism of **action it not fully understood**; however, it is believed that toxins such as chemotherapy agents cause a release of 5-HT in the gastrointestinal tract. This binds to 5-HT$_3$ receptors within the small intestine. These transmit neural impulses to the vomiting centre within the brain. The way 5-HT$_3$ receptor antagonists work to prevent postoperative nausea and vomiting is less well understood. However, the vomiting centre of the brain also receives inputs from the chemoreceptor trigger zone (CTZ), which has a high density of 5-HT$_3$ receptors. It is likely that ondansetron has **central and peripheral actions** in most children.
Clearance	Ondansetron is metabolized in the liver by multiple cytochrome P450 enzymes, namely CYP3A4, CYP2D6 and CYP1A2. A very small amount of ondansetron is excreted unchanged by the kidney. It has a **half-life of around 3–6 hours**. Liver dysfunction significantly reduces clearance and extends the half-life. Certain enzyme inducers such as phenytoin, carbamazepine and rifampicin may increase ondansetron clearance.
Administration	When given with a cycle of chemotherapy, the first dose should be immediately before chemotherapy as an intravenous (IV) dose over 15 minutes. This can subsequently be followed on with oral ondansetron. When given for the prevention of postoperative nausea and vomiting, ondansetron can be given before, during or after anaesthesia.

PRACTICAL PRESCRIBING

Dosing	Recommended dosing of ondansetron for children, from 6 months of age, is based on weight or body surface area depending on indication. The maximum daily dose of ondansetron is 32 mg. Prevention of postoperative nausea and vomiting 100 micrograms (mcg)/kg (max. 4 mg) IV over at least 30 seconds. Prevention and treatment of chemotherapy- and radiotherapy-induced nausea and vomiting (initial IV dose before commencing chemotherapy)

Body surface area	Option 1	Option 2
Up to 1.3 m²	5 mg/m² for 1 dose then give orally (see below)	150 mcg/kg (max. 8 mg/dose) repeat every 4 h for a further 2 doses before oral follow-on dose
1. 3 m² and above	8 mg for 1 dose then give orally (see below)	150 mcg/kg (max. 8 mg/dose) repeat every 4 h for a further 2 doses before oral follow-on dose

Oral follow-on doses to be commenced 12 h after IV dose for maximum 5 days

Body surface area:
Up to 0.6 m² – 2 mg every 12 h
0.6–1.2 m² – 4 mg every 12 h
1.3 m² and above – 8 mg every 12 h

OR

Weight:
Up to 10.1 kg – 2 mg every 12 h
10.1–40 kg – 4 mg every 12 h
41 kg and above – 8 mg every 12 h

Drug errors and safety	Ondansetron causes a **dose-related prolongation of the QT interval**; therefore, caution needs to be taken in any patient with potential electrolyte disorders or with cardiotoxic drugs. In view of its effect on the QT interval, congenital prolonged QT syndrome is a contraindication of ondansetron. Overdoses in the majority of cases only cause dose-related side effects such as visual disturbance, constipation, hypotension and vasovagal stimulation. Management is supportive and symptoms are often transient.
Cost	The cost has fallen considerably in the last few years. **Tablets** are now **relatively cheap**, but oral solutions, orodispersible and IV forms are still relatively expensive. Tablets cost around £1.86 for 30 × 4 mg tablets and £1.73 for 10 × 8 mg tablets. Orodispersible films are marginally cheaper than orodipsersible tablets and cost £28.50 for 10 × 4 mg films and £57 for 10 × 8 mg films. Oral solution (4 mg/5 mL) is the most expensive per dose at £38.22 for 50 mL. Solution for injection costs £29.97 for 5 vials of 4 mg/2 mL solution and £59.95 for 5 vials of 8 mg/4 mL solution.

Oxybutynin hydrochloride

CLINICAL PHARMACOLOGY

Why and when?	Oxybutynin is used in children for nocturnal enuresis associated with **overactive bladder** and to help with children who suffer from urinary frequency, urinary urgency, urinary incontinence or neurogenic bladder instability. In the context of nocturnal enuresis it may be used in conjunction with desmopressin after initial non-pharmacological treatments such as reviewing fluid intake and toileting behaviour, reward systems and enuresis alarms.
Absorption	The immediate-release form of the drug is **absorbed poorly but rapidly** reaching a maximum plasma concentration within an hour. The absolute bioavailability of oxybutynin is reported to be about 6% for the tablet form. However, there is very significant inter-individual variability in absorption. Data suggests that co-administration with food in the solution form causes a slight delay in absorption but increases bioavailability by about 25%.
Biology	Oxybutynin is a **muscarinic receptor antagonist,** acting on M_1, M_2 and M_3 receptors. It blocks the effects of parasympathetic nerve activity but appears to have a greater effect on contractions of the bladder than its other anticholinergic effects. Oxybutynin lacks receptor selectivity but **acts preferentially on the bladder** to inhibit micturition by inhibiting the muscarinic effects of acetylcholine on smooth muscle and by having a direct antispasmodic on smooth muscle. It significantly reduces sweat production in some individuals.
Clearance	It is metabolized by the cytochrome P450 enzyme systems, mostly in the liver, and is then excreted predominantly in the urine. It has a half-life of 2–3 hours. During repeated oral administration **steady state is reached after a week** of treatment.

PRACTICAL PRESCRIBING

Dosing	Dose depends upon age and whether an immediate-release or modified-release form is prescribed. Doses **need to be adjusted based upon clinical response and side effects**. Care should be taken to ensure that the smallest possible dose to achieve the desired clinical effect is prescribed. Steady-state levels take at least a week to achieve so dose increases should only be undertaken slowly.
	For nocturnal enuresis in children 5–17 years, an immediate-release medicine would be started at 2.5–3 mg twice daily which could be increased a dose of 5 mg three times a day in children <12 years and 5 mg four times a day in older children and adults if required. The last dose should be taken just prior to bedtime. Modified-release forms would be started at 5 mg once daily and adjusted in steps of 5 mg every week to maximum of 15 mg per day.
Administration	The oral format comes in immediate-release and modified-release forms. Modified-release tablets are available in 5 mg and 10 mg, immediate-release as 2.5 mg, 3 mg and 5 mg. Oral solution has two strengths – 500 micrograms per 1 mL and 1 mg per mL. When being used for neurogenic bladders it can also be administered by intravesical instillation. It is not licensed for use in children <5 years.
Drug errors and safety	Due to the rather non-selective mechanism of action, side effects are **very common**. Clinical studies involving adults report adverse reactions in **more than half** of participants. Most side effects are antimuscarinic including constipation, dry mouth, photophobia and dilation of pupils, dry skin, bradycardia and urinary retention. Oxybutynin is contraindicated in those with myasthenia gravis, conditions with significant reduced gut motility (such as gastrointestinal obstruction, paralytic ileus, pyloric stenosis and severe ulcerative colitis), porphyria and significant bladder outflow obstruction or urinary retention. There are several other medications with antimuscarinic effects (e.g. hyoscine, ipratropium) and concurrent use of two or more might increase the risk of unwanted effects occurring. Care should be taken to avoid medication errors as **two different strengths of liquid** formulations are available.
Monitoring	The **need for treatment should be reviewed** soon after commencing and at regular intervals. A response usually occurs within 6 months but may take longer.
Cost	Modified-release tablets are available at £13.77 for a pack of 28 5 mg tablets. Immediate-release tablets area available at a cost of £7.71 for a pack of 84 2.5 mg tablets. **Oral solution is more expensive** with 150 mL of 2.5 mg/5 mL costing £144.50.

Paracetamol

CLINICAL PHARMACOLOGY

Why and when?	Paracetamol (internationally known as acetaminophen) is the most common medicine encountered in paediatric practice. It is useful as an **analgesic** and **antipyretic**. Its effects are complementary with other analgesics. It can be used in children of all ages, although its biology and clearance vary by age. Its short-term safety and efficacy are well established and oral paracetamol in liquid and tablet form is available for purchase over the counter in most countries. Intravenous and rectal formulations are available for hospital use.
Absorption	Oral formulations have high bioavailability and around 80% of a dose is absorbed, mainly by passive diffusion. Absorption through the gastric mucosa **is negligible** and therefore processes or diseases that delay gastric emptying will slow absorption of oral doses. The usual time to peak blood levels after oral administration of the drug in children (aged 6 months–12 years) ranges from 0.5 to 1.8 hours and is broadly similar to adults. The presence of food delays the time to peak concentration in the blood but the overall extent of absorption is unchanged whether food is present or not. Slower gastric emptying time may delay onset of action in neonates. Rectal formulations have a reduced bioavailability compared with other routes and require higher doses to produce similar effects. Intravenous (IV) paracetamol can be helpful if gastric emptying is delayed or if a rapid onset of action is required.
Biology	Its mechanism of action is not fully understood but it is known to weakly **inhibit prostaglandin synthesis** and is highly selective for **cyclooxygenase** enzymes in the central nervous system. It also has a weak anti-inflammatory action. Paracetamol is widely distributed in the body throughout the majority of body fluids. Its analgesic activity is dependent upon penetration into the brain. It rapidly crosses the blood–brain barrier to the central nervous system with levels peaking in the cerebrospinal fluid in children after just less than 1 hour when administered intravenously.
	The clinical effects of oral paracetamol suspension in children often appear to be very rapid in clinical practice and there is probably some additional, almost immediate **placebo effect** in most children who associate the taste with feeling better. Fever responds quickly though and it typically takes just over 1 hour to resolve fever in febrile children.
Clearance	Paracetamol is primarily metabolized in **the liver** to glucuronide and sulfate conjugates that are then excreted **renally**. The **sulfation** pathway predominates **in neonates**; the **glucuronidation** pathway takes time to develop and is mature at around **2 years of age**. The elimination **half-life** for paracetamol varies between neonates, infants, children and adolescents. In neonates born at term it is between **2.5 and 4 hours**, this is about 1 hour longer than older children.

PRACTICAL PRESCRIBING

Dosing	Age- and weight-banded dosing regimens exist. Most paediatricians prefer weight-based dosing as this facilitates safe use of higher doses in most children. **Antipyretic effects** are usually achieved at **10–15 mg/kg** doses. Higher **20 mg/kg doses** may be helpful in achieving adequate **analgesia** but the maximum, safe daily dose is 75 mg/kg. The predicted half-life suggests that any effects will significantly wane after 3–4 hours in older children but after 5–6 hours in infants. Dosing regimens are therefore usually 4–6-hourly but depend upon the effect desired. The use of **antipyretic medications** to achieve a reduction of temperature in children with febrile illness is a controversial area. High temperatures in children cause parental anxiety and commonly seek medical attention. Undue emphasis on a need for reduction of fever in children has led to possible overuse of paracetamol and ibuprofen, often in combination. **There is no evidence that this reduces morbidity or mortality**.
Administration	Oral paracetamol is **widely available in a range of formulations and concentrations**. These include 120 mg/5 mL and 250 mg/5 mL suspensions, which are available over the counter and 500 mg/5 mL as a prescription-only medicine. It is available in rectal and intravenous forms and for all forms the **maximum daily dose is 75 mg/kg**. There remains debate about whether prescribers should use weight or age to determine the appropriate dose of paracetamol and the BNF-C has varied this advice over recent years. Children who are underweight or overweight for their age are at risk of receiving inappropriate doses of paracetamol.
Drug errors and safety	Prescribers and carers should beware of the potential for **accidental overdosage** and should ensure that the appropriate strength of product is prescribed (**there are several** available). Paracetamol overdose, due to medication errors, is one of the leading causes of **acute liver failure** in children. It is important to recall that many analgesic products may also contain paracetamol and cannot be used safely in combination, e.g. co-codamol, co-proxamol, many cough and flu remedies. It is important to check that these are not also being used or prescribed elsewhere on any chart. Parents should be advised to use **syringes rather than spoons** to measure the volume delivered.
Monitoring	The **efficacy** of paracetamol is measured by **serial assessment of temperature** and the use of age-appropriate **pain scoring systems**. Following overdose it is important to measure serum levels to determine the need for further monitoring and the use of acetylcysteine.
Cost	**IV** paracetamol was historically rather **expensive**, but reductions in cost coupled with improved understanding of the mechanism of action have seen an increase in its use, particularly in postoperative care where gastric emptying may be delayed. It is still more expensive than oral paracetamol costing £1.25 for 1 g compared with 2p for 1 g tablets and 15p for 1 g of oral suspension.

Paraldehyde

CLINICAL PHARMACOLOGY

Why and when?	Paraldehyde is used in the treatment of epileptic seizures, specifically to terminate **status epilepticus**. It is not commonly used as a first-line agent but is in some children who experience respiratory depression following administration of benzodiazepines. It is usually used to treat status epilepticus after benzodiazepines and/or administration of phenytoin.
Absorption	The **absorption of paraldehyde per rectum is high**, being more than 80% in most studies. Oral absorption is higher (>90%) but it is not recommended for oral use. Maximum serum concentrations are reached 30–60 minutes after administration. It is **lipid soluble** and is rapidly distributed throughout body tissues. Cerebrospinal fluid concentration is approximately 75% of serum levels.

Administration is very important. Parents and carers need to be trained to administer paraldehyde if it is prescribed for use at home. A helpful guide for parents can be found at: https://www.medicinesforchildren.org.uk/paraldehyde-seizures.

Biology	Paraldehyde has been used as a hypnotic, antiepileptic and sedative since 1882 in the UK; however, its use is now largely superseded. Despite this long history, **the exact mechanism of action is not understood**. Paraldehyde is the cyclic trimer of acetaldehyde molecules. As such is highly lipid soluble, offering excellent central nervous system (CNS) penetration, and the mechanism whereby it terminates seizures is thought to involve reduction in the amount of acetylcholine released in response to neuronal depolarization.
Clearance	A proportion of paraldehyde will be exhaled unaltered through the lungs. **An odour of paraldehyde on the breath is expected after administration**, and parents should be informed of this. Most paraldehyde is depolymerized in the liver to aldehyde, which is then oxidized by aldehyde dehydrogenase to acetic acid. This is metabolized to carbon dioxide and water, which are excreted via the lungs and kidneys, respectively. **The half-life** of paraldehyde is 3.5–9 hours, with an average of approximately **7.5 hours**.

PRACTICAL PRESCRIBING

Dosing	Dosing for neonates and children is 0.8 mL/kg (max. per dose 20 mL) for a single dose. **This is based on a solution of equal parts of paraldehyde and olive oil**.
Administration	Paraldehyde is available only in liquid form. It is a colourless liquid with a characteristic smell, supplied pre-mixed with equal volumes of olive oil. It is administered per rectum, using a plastic syringe. It is important to tell parents that **paraldehyde must be administered within 15 minutes of being drawn into the plastic syringe**, as paraldehyde degrades plastic.
	Paraldehyde also **degrades when exposed to air**, decomposing to acetaldehyde and thereafter oxidizing to acetic acid (vinegar). If on opening a bottle of paraldehyde the sharp odour of acetic acid is present, it should be discarded.
Drug errors and safety	Neat paraldehyde can cause burns to rectal mucosa; therefore, it is supplied pre-mixed in an equal volume of olive oil. **Paraldehyde should not be administered undiluted**. If consumed orally it has an unpleasant, burning taste. It can cause skin and eye irritation.
	Paraldehyde is flammable in both the liquid and vapour forms.
	In the dose recommended and used in single doses, paraldehyde is normally both safe and effective. The only commonly occurring side effect is a rash around the anus post-administration. However, paraldehyde is a CNS depressant and overdosage can result in unconsciousness and coma. Other possible effects in overdosage include headache, nausea, drowsiness, hypotension, respiratory depression and pulmonary oedema. Chronic use is dependence forming and withdrawal can cause hallucinations and convulsions.
Monitoring	As paraldehyde is normally only administered in single doses during status epilepticus, long-term dose monitoring is not required.
Cost	Paraldehyde is available as a 'special order' medication and the cost varies, but it is usually available for £9.00–10.00 for a 30 mL bottle pre-diluted in olive oil.

Phosphate (enema and supplements)

CLINICAL PHARMACOLOGY

Why and when?	Phosphate is an important, biologically relevant anion. Phosphate enemas have been in use for many decades as a laxative in refractory faecal impaction, seen in patients with **chronic constipation resistant to standard oral treatments**. Phosphate enemas are also used as part of a **bowel cleansing** regimen in preparing the colon for surgery, X-ray or endoscopic examination. It contains sodium acid phosphate and sodium phosphate. **Oral phosphate** is also fairly commonly used in children. Oral supplementation is required for children with low serum phosphate (0.5–0.9 mmol/L). Children with very low serum phosphate levels (<0.5 mmol/L) often require **intravenous (IV) phosphate boluses**. Levels below 0.3 mmol/L are life-threatening. Commoner reasons for hypophosphataemia include **preterm neonates** who have low stores and higher requirements and hypophosphataemia during **refeeding syndrome**, which occurs when adequate nutrition is started after a period of prolonged starvation.
Absorption and distribution	Colonic absorption of phosphate following rectal administration is probably minimal. Mostly because it acts quickly, leading to bowel evacuation **within 5–10 minutes** in most children. Oral phosphate is absorbed mostly in the small intestine via an active, energy-dependent process. In adults about **two-thirds of oral phosphate is absorbed**. Foods or drugs containing large amounts of calcium or aluminium decrease phosphate absorption but it is enhanced when phosphate and calcium are administered in equal amounts (as in milk). Phosphate absorption is also stimulated by vitamin D. Total body phosphate is **very unequally distributed** between body compartments. 85% is bound in the hydroxyapatite matrix of bone. Of the remaining 15% almost all is intracellular. It is the most abundant intracellular anion but the **free intracellular concentration is only about 10 mmol/L**. This is still 10 times higher than the extracellular concentration which is around 1 mmol/L. Phosphate is actively transported into cells by an insulin-activated sodium-phosphate co-transporter.
Biology	Phosphate is **essential for glucose metabolism** and **bone mineralization**. The shift to glucose metabolism during refeeding results in a high demand for phosphorylated intermediates required for glycolysis, the Krebs cycle, and to form adenosine triphosphate and 2,3-diphosphoglycerate. This results in a **reduction in serum phosphate levels**. Its mechanism of action as an enema is not well understood. Its laxative action may result from the osmotic activity of the sodium acid phosphate. Fluid accumulation in the stool produces rectal distension and promotes bowel peristalsis.
Clearance	Phosphate forms part of the glomerular ultrafiltrate and in adults about 7 g is filtered per day and 85–90% is **actively reabsorbed**. Its excretion is diminished in renal failure and must be used with caution in patients with impaired renal function. During periods of growth and active bone mineralization extracellular phosphate will be actively transported into cells and bones.

PRACTICAL PRESCRIBING

Dosing and administration	**Prevention of hypophosphataemia in 34-week gestation babies taking unsupplemented breast milk:** <0.5 mmol/kg 3 times a day until 36–44 weeks corrected gestational age.

Dosing and administration

Prevention of hypophosphataemia in 34-week gestation babies taking unsupplemented breast milk:
<0.5 mmol/kg 3 times a day until 36–44 weeks corrected gestational age.

Treatment of moderate hypophosphataemia (oral preparations):
Neonate: 1 mmol/kg daily in 1–2 divided doses. Child 1 month– 4 years: 2–3 mmol/kg daily in 2–4 divided doses (max. initial dose 48 mmol/day). Child 5–17 years: 2–3 mmol/kg/daily in 2–4 divided doses (max. initial dose 96 mmol/day). Adjust doses as necessary according to serum levels.

Phosphate is available in two oral forms: effervescent tablets, Phosphate-Sandoz® (each tablet contains 16.1 mmol phosphate, 20.4 mmol sodium and 3.1 mmol potassium) and liquid forms, Joulies phosphate. Joulies solution contains 1 mmol phosphate and 0.76 mmol sodium per mL.

As bowel preparation:
Child 3–6 years: 45–65 mL once daily. Child 7–11 years 65–100 mL once daily. Child 12–17 years 100–128 mL once daily.

Side effects and interactions

Following oral administration **diarrhoea is a common side effect** and may require dosage to be reduced. Phosphate depletion occurs in severe diabetic ketoacidosis. Insulin infusions will lower serum levels by increasing active transport into cells. If a phosphate enema is retained then hyperphosphataemia may occur.

Infant formula and breast milk fortifiers also contain relatively high amounts of phosphate. The total phosphate load (intake) should be calculated in these babies prior to supplementation.

Monitoring

Children at risk for refeeding syndrome should have baseline serum electrolytes including serum phosphate checked. Individuals with low baseline levels require very regular (at least daily) monitoring and some centres will consider using oral phosphate early as there is likely to be a fall in serum phosphate within 48 hours of restoring a positive energy balance. It is usual practice to also undertake and ECG and **look for evidence of prolongation of the QT interval**.

The efficacy of phosphate enema is measured by the stool output.

Cost

Tablets are relatively cheap. Each Phosphate-Sandoz tablet costs about 20p. Joulies phosphate is **expensive** and considered as a high-cost medicine.

Piperacillin with tazobactam (Tazocin®)

CLINICAL PHARMACOLOGY

Why and when?	Piperacillin and tazobactam are often used in combination. Tazocin® is a branded combination of these products, which are now available in generic forms. The combination of a penicillin, in this case a ureidopenicillin, with a β-lactamase inhibitor **increases its spectrum of antimicrobial activity**. It is **bactericidal**. Piperacillin and tazobactam combination is effective against a range of Gram-positive and Gram-negative bacteria as well as anaerobes. **It is not active against methicillin-resistant *Staphylococcus aureus* (MRSA)**. It is specifically used in hospital-acquired pneumonia, septicaemia, skin, urinary tract, soft tissue and intra-abdominal bacterial infections. It has an important place in the treatment of children **with neutropenia** (low total neutrophil count) and **possible infection** (fever) where it is used first line by many UK centres.
Absorption	Tazocin is not orally absorbed. It is given via intravenous (IV) infusion. Tazocin moderately (30%) binds to plasma proteins. The remaining 70% **distributes well into most tissues and crosses the blood–brain barrier**. Typical minimum inhibitory concentrations (MICs) are low. They range between 0.06 and 16 micrograms (mcg)/mL depending on the bacteria being treated. The tissue concentrations achieved are usually much higher. After a 4 g/0.5 g dose, the peak tissue concentration in adults is 298 mcg/mL (piperacillin) and 34 mcg/mL (tazobactam), respectively.
Biology	**Piperacillin** is an **extended-spectrum penicillin** antibiotic that is already somewhat resistant to degradation by β-lactamases. **Tazobactam** further **inhibits β-lactamase** and prevents the destruction of piperacillin. Piperacillin kills bacteria by inhibiting the synthesis of bacterial cell walls. It binds preferentially to specific penicillin-binding proteins (PBPs) located inside bacterial cell walls. PBPs vary among bacterial species, and thus susceptibility to piperacillin depends on the ability of piperacillin to bind to the specific PBPs of each species.
	Susceptible bacteria include:
	❶ Aerobic and facultative Gram-positive microorganisms, e.g. *Staphylococcus aureus*.
	❷ Aerobic and facultative Gram-negative microorganisms, e.g. *Escherichia coli*, *Haemophilus influenzae*, *Klebsiella pneumoniae* and *Pseudomonas aeruginosa*.
	❸ Gram-negative anaerobes, e.g. *Bacteroides fragilis* group.
Clearance	Piperacillin and tazobactam both have **short half-lives**, between **0.6 and 1.2 hours**. The dosing is usually every 8 hours but can be shortened to 6-hourly to ensure the MIC is maintained at a bactericidal level. Piperacillin and tazobactam are eliminated **primarily by the kidney**; they are excreted rapidly as unchanged drug in high concentrations in the urine. They are also excreted in the bile and can be used safely in children with severely restricted kidney function, although the half-life may increase to 8 hours in acute renal failure.

PRACTICAL PRESCRIBING

Dosing	Dosing is dependent on the child's age and weight as well as the indication for use. It is licensed for children over 2 years of age with neutropenia or complicated abdominal infections (see Table below).
Administration	Piperacillin with tazobactam can only be given intravenously. For IV infusion, dilute the reconstituted solution to a concentration of 15–90 mg/mL with either glucose 5% or sodium chloride 0.9% solutions and give over 30 minutes.
Drug errors and safety	Piperacillin and tazobactam is usually well tolerated with few side effects. In common with many antibiotics it may result in hypersensitivity reactions. **It should be avoided in children with known penicillin allergy.** High doses worsen hypernatraemia. Each vial of Tazocin 2 g/0.25 g contains 5.67 mmol (130 mg) of sodium. Under some circumstances it produces a false-positive urinary glucose (if tested for reducing substances).
Monitoring	Routine monitoring of serum levels is not required.
Cost	Piperacillin/tazobactam combination is **relatively expensive**. Currently 2 g/250 mg dose for 10 vials costs up to £60 with individual vials costing £9.70. The 4 g/500 mg dose per vial can cost between £12 and £20.

Dose dependant on age as well as treatment time frame

Condition	Dose			
	Neonate	1 month–11 years	2–11 years	12–17 years
Hospital-acquired pneumonia, septicaemia, complicated urinary tract/skin/soft tissue infections	90 mg/kg every 8 h	90 mg/kg every 6–8 h (max. per dose 4.5 g every 6 h)	–	4.5 g every 8 h; severe infection increased if necessary to 4.5 g every 6 h
Complicated abdominal infections			112.5 mg/kg every 8 h (max. per dose 4.5 g)	4.5 g every 8 h; severe infection increased if necessary to 4.5 g every 6 h
Infections in neutropenic patients	90 mg/kg every 6 h (max. per dose 4.5 g)			

Prednisolone

CLINICAL PHARMACOLOGY

Why and when?	Prednisolone is a potent **synthetic corticosteroid** used to **reduce inflammation and suppress the immune system**. It has a mainly glucocorticoid effect with some very limited mineralocorticoid effects (see Appendix 3 for comparative potencies of commonly used steroids). It is used to treat a wide range of allergic, autoimmune, inflammatory and malignant conditions. It is commonly used in children to treat **exacerbations of asthma**. It is used in high doses to treat **nephrotic syndrome** and can be used in lower doses to maintain control. It is available as tablets, eye and ear drops and as either rectal foam or suppositories.
Absorption	Under most circumstances, prednisolone is readily absorbed from the gastrointestinal (GI) tract with a **bioavailability of approximately 70%**. Absorption is reduced in some conditions when enteric-coated tablets are used and these should not be used in children with **cystic fibrosis**. Peak plasma concentration is reached **1–2 hours after administration** of non-enteric-coated oral prednisolone and **2–3 hours after enteric-coated tablets**. Prednisolone is >90% plasma bound. The majority is to a specific protein, **corticosteroid-binding globulin**, and the remainder to albumin. Hypoalbuminaemia increases the proportion of unbound drug and can therefore increase adverse effects. Prednisolone crosses the blood–brain barrier and the placenta. Small amounts are also excreted in breast milk.
Biology	Prednisolone enters the cell and forms a complex by combining **with intracellular glucocorticoid receptors**. The complex enters the cell nucleus and binds to the promoter region of the target genes controlling the synthesis of certain proteins including enzymes that regulate many metabolic functions such as inflammation. One key enzyme that is inhibited is **phospholipase A2**, which is involved in the formation of arachidonic acid and inflammatory mediators.
Clearance and relative potencies of steroids	Prednisolone is mostly **metabolized by the liver** to a biologically inactive compound. The half-life of prednisolone is increased by liver disease. A small proportion (c.5%) is excreted unchanged in the urine. The plasma half-life (time for the blood plasma concentration to halve) of prednisolone is only 3–4 hours but the biological half-life (time for the activity of a drug to lose one half its initial effectiveness) is 18–36 hours, meaning it is appropriate for daily or alternate day administration. The half-life of prednisolone is **usually shorter in younger children**.

PRACTICAL PRESCRIBING

Dosing	For most indications there is academic debate about the best dose. The maximum oral dose recommended for children is in **nephrotic syndrome: 60 mg/m^2 once daily (max. 80 mg)**. In asthma and croup it is usual to give **1–2 mg/kg to a maximum of 40 mg daily** but in life-threatening or severe episodes doses up to 60 mg are sometimes used. Due to its extended duration of action it is nearly always given **once daily**. It is given more frequently (6-hourly initially) in the initial treatment of **infantile spasms**. The length of course depends upon the indication and likely pathophysiology. In croup it is usually given once daily for 3 days, in asthma 3–7 days, and in nephrotic syndrome for several weeks.
Administration	Oral enteric-coated tablets should be **swallowed without chewing** with milk, juice or water. For children too young to swallow whole tablets the non-enteric-coated tablets can be **crushed and mixed with soft food,** i.e. yogurt or jam. Sweet food works better as the tablets have a bitter taste and the child needs to swallow without chewing if possible. Soluble tablets should be **dissolved in water or fruit cordial**. They are also bitter and sweet fruit cordials often help to partially mask the taste. A syringe can be helpful. **If a child vomits within 30 minutes** of a dose, a **repeat dose** should be given. After 30 minutes repeat dosing is usually not required.
Side effects and Interactions	Side effects **are common** even with short courses and include gastritis (particularly with non-enteric-coated prednisolone), hyperglycaemia, increased appetite and hyperactivity or mood disturbances. More rarely, serious side effects, including upper GI ulceration, glaucoma or impaired clotting, may occur. In common with all steroids, continuous use at doses higher than natural production will suppress endogenous production. Gradual withdrawal (tapering and weaning) should be considered in those who have received **more than 40 mg of prednisolone for a week**, in those who have been given **repeated doses in the evening** or in children who have received **more than 3 weeks' treatment**.
Monitoring	**Growth should be monitored** in children who are receiving either long-term treatment with prednisolone or those who are receiving frequent oral steroid bursts. Children who have required long courses of treatment should have screening for bone density (DEXA scanning).
Cost	Most **tablets are cheap**. As they are commonly used this is an important consideration. 5 mg tablets are typically 3–4p each. Soluble tablets are significantly more costly and, depending on the manufacturer, they cost 50p–£2 per 5 mg tablet. Prednisolone foam for local treatment of colonic bowel inflammation is more expensive, costing c.£13 per enema.

Propranolol

CLINICAL PHARMACOLOGY

Why and when?	Propranolol is a **non-selective β-blocker** without intrinsic sympathomimetic activity. It is a competitive antagonist of β_1-adrenoceptors (located in the heart) and β_2-adrenoceptors (located in peripheral vasculature, bronchi, pancreas, liver and skeletal muscle). **It has a wide range of clinical indications** including treatment of arrhythmias, hypertension, prevention and treatment of cyanotic spells associated with tetralogy of Fallot, thyrotoxicosis and migraine prophylaxis. It has recently demonstrated significant efficacy in the treatment of proliferating infantile haemangioma.
Absorption and distribution	Oral doses of propranolol are fully absorbed with plasma concentrations peaking 1–2 hours post administration. Despite the good enteral absorption, there is **significant first-pass metabolism** in the liver leading to a **much lower effective bioavailability of about 25%**. The majority is protein bound. Propranolol is distributed rapidly throughout the body and as it is **lipid soluble** it rapidly crosses the blood–brain barrier. After administration, the highest concentrations are found in the lungs, liver, kidney, brain and heart.
Biology	Propranolol is a racemic compound. This means is contains equal amounts of left- and right-handed optical isomers. The L-isomer is the active version. It **competes with neurotransmitters such as catecholamines for binding at adrenergic receptors inhibiting sympathetic stimulation**. The action of propranolol in blocking β_1-adrenoceptors slows heart rate and atrioventricular node conduction as well as reducing cardiac contractility. These negative inotropic effects cause a fall in cardiac output. Its action in blocking β_2-adrenoceptors causes bronchoconstriction, peripheral vasoconstriction and metabolic imbalances including hypoglycaemia, hyperglycaemia and hypertriglyceridemia. It also significantly impairs the effectiveness of bronchodilators such as salbutamol. Propranolol also affects the metabolism of thyroxine by **inhibiting the conversion of T_4 to the more potent T_3 hormone**. Excess T_4 is converted to reverse T_3 which is inactive.
	The action of propranolol in treating infantile haemangioma is not known. It is probably mediated through a combination of effects including **reduced blood flow**, an indirect action reducing **vascular endothelial growth factor** production (VEGF) and **increased apoptosis**.
Clearance	When administered orally, 90% is removed by the liver with an **elimination half-life of 3–4 hours**. The main metabolite 4-hydroxypropranolol, with a longer half-life (5–7.5 h) than the parent compound (3–4 h), is also pharmacologically active. The plasma half-life of IV propranolol is approximately 2 hours.

PRACTICAL PRESCRIBING

Dosing	The dosing regimen varies widely depending on the indication. Expert guidance should be sought for treatment of infantile haemangioma, arrhythmias or management of tetralogy of Fallot. Hyperthyroidism, thyrotoxicosis and thyrotoxic crisis Neonate: 250–500 micrograms (mcg)/kg orally (or 20–50 mcg/kg IV) every 6–8 hours adjusted according to response. Child: 250–500 mcg/kg every 8 hours (or 25–50 mcg/kg IV every 6–8 hours) adjusted according to response (up to 1 mg/kg). Maximum IV dose 5 mg and maximum oral dose 40 mg. Hypertension Neonate: 250 mcg/kg orally 3 times a day increased up to 2 mg/kg 8-hourly. Child: 0.25–1 mg/kg orally 3 times a day, increased as necessary at weekly intervals to 5 mg/kg/day in divided doses. Older children (12–17 years): 80 mg twice daily increased weekly as necessary up to 320 mg/day. Migraine prophylaxis Child 2–11 years: 200–500 mcg/kg twice daily; usual dose 10–20 mg twice daily. Older children (12–17 years): 20–40 mg twice daily initially; usual dose 40–80 mg twice daily.
Administration	Propranolol is usually administered **by mouth 2–3 times per day**. It can be given intravenously to treat toxic hyperthyroid states, severe cyanotic spells in children with tetralogy of Fallot and arrhythmias. Oral solution is available in a range of concentrations.
Side effects and errors	Blockage of β_1-adrenoceptors can cause **bradycardia and hypotension**. Its negative inotropic effects mean its use is contraindicated in children with second- or third-degree heart block. Blockage of β_2-adrenoceptors in the lungs and peripheral vasculature can cause bronchoconstriction resulting in exacerbations of asthma and peripheral vasoconstriction causing Raynaud's phenomenon. **It is contraindicated in individuals with asthma**. Oral solutions come in a range of concentrations from 1 mg/mL to 10 mg/mL. **Very great care must be taken to ensure that concentrations are not changed without very careful discussion with families**.
Monitoring	Children receiving IV propranolol should have continuous ECG monitoring.
Cost	Propranolol is **relatively cheap**. Tablets come in sizes of 10 mg, 40 mg, 80 mg and 160 mg and cost 5–6p each. Modified-release preparations of 80 mg or 160 mg capsules are only slightly more expensive and may allow once-daily dosing. Oral solution is considerably more expensive costing between £12.5 and £20 for 150 mL of the oral solution (available in various concentrations).

Ranitidine

CLINICAL PHARMACOLOGY

Why and when?	Ranitidine is mainly used to treat **moderate-to-severe gastro-oesophageal reflux disease** (GORD). Oral preparations are unlicensed for children under 3 years and the injection is unlicensed for children under 6 months. It is generally **well tolerated** and short-term efficacy is proven with limited evidence of long-term effects on growth and development. In children it can also be used as prophylaxis to reduce the frequency of acute bleeding in oesophageal varices and prevention of degradation of pancreatic enzyme supplements in cystic fibrosis (CF) patients.
Absorption	Orally administered ranitidine undergoes significant first pass hepatic metabolism and it has a **bioavailability of around 50%**. It has a rapid and peak plasma concentration usually achieved 2–3 hours after oral administration. Oral absorption is unreliable in neonates. The absorption is not affected by food or antacid use and unabsorbed ranitidine may act directly on the parietal cells within the gastric mucosa of the stomach as relief of heartburn occurs quickly in adult studies (within 30 min).
Biology	Ranitidine is a selective histamine receptor 2 (H_2) antagonist. The H_2 receptors are found on parietal cells within the gastric mucosa of the stomach. Ranitidine **competitively inhibits and blocks** the **binding of histamine** released from the gastric mucosa. This blocks basal and meal-stimulated acid (H^+) secretion via the hydrogen ion/potassium ATPase channel into the stomach lumen, increasing gastric pH. This also reduces the effect of other substances such as gastrin and acetylcholine that promote acid secretion via stimulation of H_2 receptors. Overall, **ranitidine reduces the acid and volume of gastric secretions**. Ranitidine has a long duration of action as a single 150 mg dose will supresses gastric acid for 12 hours. There are also H_2 receptors within cardiac tissue and blockade of the cardiac H_2 receptors can result in bradycardia, a very rare side effect at therapeutic doses.
Clearance	Only 15% of ranitidine is plasma protein bound and it has a large volume of distribution (1.4 L/kg). It is does not cross the blood–brain barrier but is concentrated in breast milk. Following IV use its elimination half-life is **approximately 2 hours in adults and older children** (aged 3–18). Most is cleared renally but there is some hepatic metabolism. Neonates have less predictable oral absorption but slower clearance.

PRACTICAL PRESCRIBING

Dosing

Age range	Oral dose	IV dose
Neonates (<1 month)	2 mg/kg (max. 3 mg/kg) 8-hourly	0.5–1 mg/kg every 6–8 hours
Babies (1–5 months)	1 mg/kg 8-hourly	1 mg/kg 8-hourly
Infant (6 months–3 yrs)	2–4 mg/kg 12-hourly	1 mg/kg 8-hourly
Child (3–11 yrs)	2–4 mg/kg (max 5 mg/kg) 12-hourly	1 mg/kg 8-hourly (max. 50 mg)
Older child (12–17 yrs)	150 mg 12-hourly (max. 600 mg/day)	50 mg/kg every 6–8 h

Drug errors and safety	Ranitidine is generally well tolerated with uncommon side effects including abdominal pain, constipation and nausea, which are mostly improved during continued treatment. As ranitidine is a very selective drug it is relatively safe. In overdose it can have cardiac effects but these are rare. Ranitidine can affect the bioavailability of many drugs that require an acid environment to aid absorption. **Ranitidine syrup contains alcohol** and therefore should be avoided in these patients who are at risk, especially if they have pre-existing liver disease. It may be culturally unacceptable for some families.
Administration	Ranitidine is available in tablet (75 mg, 150 mg or 300 mg), effervescent tablet (150 mg, 300 mg), oral solution (75 mg/5 mL) and intravenous (IV) forms. For IV forms it is advised to dilute the solution with either glucose 5% or sodium chloride 0.9% and give over at least 3 minutes. Rapid administration can result in bradycardia. Oral forms can be taken with or without food, but it is recommended that if it is being taken to reduce degradation of pancreatic enzyme supplements then oral doses should be given 1–2 hours before food to enhance their effects.
Monitoring	Routine monitoring of drug levels is **not required**; children who require prolonged treatment for symptomatic gastroesophageal reflux may require review by a paediatric gastroenterologist for consideration of endoscopy.
Cost	Ranitidine **tablets are relatively inexpensive** and can be purchased without prescription in the UK. 150 mg tablets cost just over 2p each. Oral solutions are slightly more expensive but still fairly cheap. The 75 mg/5 mL solution costs around 2p/mL. Effervescent tablet forms are far more expensive costing between 50p and 60p per 150 mg tablet. Intravenous forms are the most expensive. For the IV solution, 150 mg as 25 mg/mL solution costs between £2.69 and £5.

Rifampicin

CLINICAL PHARMACOLOGY

Why and when?	Rifampicin is a semi-synthetic bactericidal antibiotic produced from *Streptomyces mediterranei*. Rifampicin has a **broad spectrum of activity** against bacteria, mainly Gram-positive cocci and *Mycobacterium tuberculosis*. However, because of **rapid development of resistance** its use has been restricted. Rifampicin is most commonly used for treatment and prophylaxis of tuberculosis and for leprosy. It is also useful for elimination of *Neisseria meningococci* in carriers (but not recommended for active meningococcal infection) and for Gram-positive (*Staphylococcus aureus*, *Staph. epidermidis*, *Streptococcus pyogenes*, S. *viridans* and S. *pneumoniae*) and Gram-negative bacteria (*Haemophilus influenzae* type B). It has some anti-chlamydial activity and *in vitro* activity against some viruses (poxvirus and adenovirus) at high doses.
Absorption and distribution	Rifampicin is very well absorbed (90%) after oral administration. Co-administration with food will reduce absorption by about a third and absorption is also somewhat reduced in neonates. It is widely distributed in the body tissues and fluids including cerebrospinal fluid, so much so that it can **impart orange-red colour** to the urine, faeces, saliva, sputum, tears and sweat. Absorption may be delayed or there can be a slightly reduced peak if administered with food. It has a very high protein binding of about 80%. Peak serum concentrations occur 2–4 hours after oral administration.
Biology	Rifampicin, a semi-synthetic derivative of rifamycin, inhibits bacterial DNA-dependent ribonucleic acid (RNA) synthesis by **inhibiting bacterial DNA-dependent RNA polymerase** by forming a stable drug-enzyme complex. The corresponding mammalian enzymes are not affected by rifampicin. The inhibitor prevents RNA synthesis by physically blocking elongation, and thus preventing synthesis of host bacterial proteins. At therapeutic levels rifampicin is a **bactericidal agent.** There is a **rapid development of resistance** with rifampicin use, which hinders its widespread use. 95% of bacterial rifampicin resistance mutations are present in *rpoB gene* and molecular genetic analysis of *M. tuberculosis* isolates can determine sensitivity before culture results are available.
Clearance	Rifampicin is **rapidly eliminated in bile** and undergoes enterohepatic circulation. Its usual biological half-life is between 1.5 and 5 hours. It undergoes progressive deacetylation and almost all the drug is in this form in the bile in about 6 hours. However, this metabolite retains complete antibacterial activity. Approximately 60–65% of drug is excreted in faeces and around **30% drug is excreted in urine** (more than half of which is unchanged drug).
	Half-life elimination can be increased significantly with hepatic and renal impairment. The half-life may be decreased in patients receiving isoniazid. Rifampicin is a strong inducer of many of the CYP450 group of enzymes. It predictably results in a lot of drug interactions.

CLINICAL PHARMACOLOGY

Dosing	Rifampicin dosing is **age- and weight-dependent**. Dosage for treatment or prevention of tuberculosis is **15 mg/kg** with a maximum daily dose of 450 mg for children <50 kg and 600 mg for those >50 kg. It is **never used alone for the treatment of infections** and always in combination with other drugs to prevent development of resistance. For **brucellosis, Legionnaires' disease and serious streptococcal infections**, it is used in a dose of 5–10 mg/kg twice daily in children <1 year and 10 mg/kg twice daily in children > 1 year. Rifampicin can be used for **prophylaxis of H. influenzae type B** infection in a dose of 10 mg/kg once daily in children 1–2 months of age, 20 mg/kg once daily in children 3 months–11 years, and 600 mg once daily in children 12–17 years for a total of 4 days. For **prevention of secondary cases of meningococcal meningitis**, rifampicin is given twice daily for 2 days at 5 mg/kg for those <12 months, 10 mg/kg for those aged 1–11 years and 600 mg for older children. Whilst unlicensed for this indication, rifampicin is used **in children for pruritis due to cholestasis** in a dose of 5–10 mg/kg once daily. For all children the maximum daily dose for any indication is 600 mg (except where given under direct expert supervision for TB treatment).
Administration	Oral rifampicin should be given on **empty stomach,** either 30 minutes prior or 2 hours after a meal. It is **usually given in the morning**. Capsules should be swallowed with a glass of water or juice (but not milk) and not chewed.
Drug errors and safety	Rifampicin can commonly cause nausea, vomiting, diarrhoea, thrombocytopenia and leucopenia. Rare but **life-threatening** side effects include hypersensitivity reactions, severe cutaneous adverse reactions, toxic epidermal necrolysis, and DRESS (drug rash with eosinophilia and systemic symptoms) syndrome. Rifampicin may **permanently stain soft contact-lenses**; hence, it is important not to use them during therapy.
Monitoring	Routine monitoring of rifampicin is **not required**. Pre-treatment liver and renal function should be checked. If pre-treatment liver function is normal further checks are needed only if the patient develops symptoms.
Cost	Rifampicin is a **fairly expensive** drug. It is cheaper in the form of oral solution, the preferred form for children, where each 150 mg dose costs about 26p. However, in capsule form, each 150 mg capsule costs about 50p whilst a 300 mg capsule costs £1.23. When it is used parenterally, a form in which it is used only rarely, it costs £9.20 for a 600 mg dose. Since it is used as a part of long-term regimens, the overall cost can be very high.

Salbutamol

CLINICAL PHARMACOLOGY

Why and when?	Salbutamol is a **bronchodilator**, commonly used in paediatrics to treat **asthma and wheezing**. It is most commonly given via an inhaler with a spacer device, although nebulized and intravenous (IV) forms can also be given to treat moderate-to-severe wheeze, particularly when there is an oxygen requirement. It is rarely effective in patients under the age of 12 months of age.
Absorption	When salbutamol is nebulized, only a relatively small proportion of the dose reaches the lungs, with the remainder lost to the environment, in the mouth or the inhaler device. Typically, **inhaled routes with spacer devices result in higher (3–4-fold) proportional lung deposition** (around 20% in studies of children using spacers with masks) and therefore the doses required to achieve similar effects are much lower. Salbutamol, which reaches the lungs, is ultimately absorbed into the systemic circulation and is metabolized by the liver. Oral salbutamol solutions are available and **oral salbutamol has a bioavailability of 40–50%**. However, the use of oral salbutamol is restricted to highly specialized indications where systemic availability is desired, i.e. in children with spinal muscular atrophy type 2.
Biology	Salbutamol is a selective and **partial β_2-agonist**. It has maximum effects at relatively low doses. Stimulation of the β-2 receptors in the bronchi leads to bronchodilation. In turn this improves airway resistance in the small airways and a reduction of wheeze. The duration of action of salbutamol is typically 4–6 hours, although in patients with moderate or severe asthma or wheeze, it often needs to be given more regularly than this. The β_2-receptor is a G protein-coupled receptor that activates adenylyl cyclase, **producing cyclic adenosine monophosphate (AMP)**, leading to smooth muscle relaxation including in the bronchi. The mechanism of this is not fully understood but is thought to involve calcium and protein kinase A. Salbutamol has effects on other organs with β-2 receptors, including the heart and muscles. **Tremor and tachycardia** are common additional effects.
Clearance	**The half-life of IV salbutamol is approximately 4 hours**. Salbutamol that has been absorbed into the systemic circulation is metabolized by the liver. Metabolism occurs through the production of phenolic sulfate, which is mostly renally excreted. Salbutamol that has been absorbed through the gastrointestinal tract undergoes significant first-pass metabolism by the liver.
Administration	Whenever possible **inhaled salbutamol should be given via a spacer device** as this improves efficiency of delivery. In acute asthma and wheeze, inhaled salbutamol is usually given via pressurized metered dose inhalers, but dry powder devices are also available. Nebulized salbutamol is available in liquid vials containing 2.5 mg or 5 mg depending on the age of the child.

PRACTICAL PRESCRIBING

Dosing	Salbutamol dosing depends on the route of administration. All doses are given 'as required'.

Inhaled salbutamol dosage is 2–10 puffs (200 micrograms (mcg) − 1 mg).

Nebulized salbutamol dosage is 2.5 mg for children <5 years and 5 mg for older children.

If inhaled or nebulized salbutamol is needed as frequently as hourly following initial stabilization, alternative treatments are considered, i.e. ipratropium, magnesium or IV salbutamol or aminophylline.

IV salbutamol is prescribed based on weight and age. **Toxicity can occur at recommended doses and it should be used with caution**.

In children under 2 years, a bolus dose can be given of 5 mcg/kg over 5 minutes. In older children, the dosage is 15 mcg/kg (up to 250 mcg). This is usually followed by an infusion can also be given, of 1–5 mcg/kg/min, with careful monitoring of heart rate and potassium. **Great care must be taken in children with higher weights** and dosing in this group is controversial. Children requiring rates of >2 mcg/kg/min should be admitted to a paediatric intensive care unit. |
| Drug errors and safety | Overdosage of salbutamol is reported to be low, but side effects of this medication are common. This means that **careful monitoring is needed of children requiring frequent salbutamol**, and regular reviews to consider whether escalation is needed to alternative treatment is important.

Frequent usage of salbutamol, such as long periods of hourly inhaled or nebulized salbutamol, or requirement for IV salbutamol, can lead to side effects, particularly tachycardia, hypokalaemia and raised lactate (lactic acidosis). |
| Monitoring | The British National Formulary for Children recommends that patients being treated for severe asthma should have their plasma potassium concentration monitored. In practice, these children also have lactate levels (as part of a blood gas that also provides information about respiratory status) and heart rates monitored. Additionally, patients with diabetes should have their blood glucose monitored due to the possibility of development of hyperglycaemia and ketoacidosis. |
| Cost | Salbutamol in all forms is **relatively cheap**. Inhaled salbutamol administered via a chlorofluorocarbon-free pressured dose inhaler costs c. £1.50 for 200 doses. Dry powder devices are slightly more expensive. Nebulized salbutamol costs about 10p for 2.5 mg or 20p for a 5 mg dose; however, consumable equipment required to deliver nebulizers often adds significantly to the overall cost. IV salbutamol costs approximately 40p for a 500 mcg ampoule and £2.50 for a 5 mg ampoule. |

Salmeterol

CLINICAL PHARMACOLOGY

Why and when?	Salmeterol is used in the management of children with **chronic asthma**. Salmeterol is a long-acting β_2-agonist (LABA). It is **not effective in the management of acute exacerbations** but when used in the chronic asthma it reduces exacerbations. The place of LABA in asthma treatment guidelines for children varies and currently there are differences between different sets of national and international guidelines. In general, a LABA is trialled before higher doses of inhaled steroids are given. Salmeterol is typically used in children over the age of 5, as leukotriene receptor antagonists (LRTAs) are preferred in children under 5. It is inhaled as an aerosol or powder twice daily.

Salmeterol is a **partial agonist and has a slower onset of action than other LABAs** like formoterol, which is a full agonist. Salmeterol is therefore **not suitable for maintenance and reliever therapy** (MART) but should be used in fixed-dose regimens. The use of **LABA monotherapy** in children **is dangerous** and therefore it is almost always prescribed as a combination inhaler, i.e. combined with an inhaled steroid. |
Absorption and distribution	Salmeterol is delivered either via a pressurized metered dose inhaler (pMDI) or dry powder inhaler (DPI). When a pMDI is used then drug delivery is nearly always better if used with a **valved holding chamber** (spacer device). Most guidelines recommend the use of a pMDI with spacer as the preferred option for children with asthma. Inhaled particles with a diameter of 2–4 μm will deposit in the conducting airways and from there can act upon local β_2-receptors. Systemic levels of salmeterol **are often undetectable after inhalation of recommended doses**, probably as a result of significant first-pass metabolism.
Biology	Salmeterol is a β_2-agonist and has the same mechanism of action as short-acting β agonists such as salbutamol. **It is approximately 8 times as potent as salbutamol**. Salmeterol has a lipophilic side chain that prevents degradation, making it much longer acting; it has an 8–12-hour duration of clinical activity. Salmeterol binds to β_2 receptors on membranes of bronchial smooth muscle. Stimulation of these receptors causes a cascade of intracellular signalling: activation of Gs protein, adenylyl cyclase activation, increased intracellular levels of cAMP and activation of protein kinase A (PKA) ultimately leading to smooth muscle relaxation and bronchodilation. Mechanisms by which PKA may do this are through decreased intracellular calcium, increased membrane potassium conductance and decreased myosin light chain phosphorylation leading to smooth muscle relaxation.
Clearance	Salmeterol acts locally within the lungs. Most is not orally absorbed or cleared systemically. In adult studies just over half of the radioactivity from radiolabelled salmeterol is recovered in the faeces and about a quarter in the urine. The small amounts that do reach the systemic circulation are subject to inactivation by the CYP3A4 enzymes. The systemic **half-life in adults is 12–15 hours**.

PRACTICAL PRESCRIBING

Dosing	Salmeterol is only licensed in children from 5 years of age. **The usual dose is 50 micrograms (mcg) twice daily**. Whilst higher doses (up to 100 mcg twice daily) have been used in adults and older children (12–17 years), these are not recommended by most clinicians.
Administration	Salmeterol is usually given twice each day, once in the morning and once in the evening. Ideally, these times are 10–12 hours apart. **A valved holding chamber (spacer) should be used if a pMDI is used**. It is also available as a DPI. DPIs require a higher inspiratory flow rate and are **usually not suitable for younger children**. Regardless of the inhaler type prescribed, training in its use must be given to the child and the family. Errors in technique are common and **inhaler technique should be reviewed regularly**.
Side effects and interactions	The side effects are **similar to those seen for salbutamol**. Common side effects of salmeterol include arrhythmias, dizziness, headaches, nausea, muscle cramps, palpitations and tremor. High doses can be associated with hypokalaemia. There are no absolute contraindications with salmeterol; however, some medications are thought to increase the risk of hypokalaemia and should be used with caution or avoided where possible. These include antifungals such as ketoconazole, clarithromycin, some selective serotonin reuptake inhibitors (SSRIs) and numerous other medications. Use of salmeterol alongside digoxin may increase risk of digoxin toxicity.
Monitoring and safety	Under normal circumstances and when recommended doses are used, **monitoring is not required**. **Salmeterol should never be used without an inhaled corticosteroid**. If it is used as monotherapy for treatment of asthma, there is an increased risk of death. It is therefore safer to only prescribe this in forms that are combined with inhaled steroids. These are often cheaper.
Cost	Salmeterol is **fairly expensive,** particularly if prescribed as a separate inhaler. 25 mcg dose inhalers cost about £30 for 120 doses (i.e. 1 month's supply). **It is cheaper when prescribed as a combination inhaler**. A salmeterol 25 mcg/fluticasone 50 mcg combination pMDI costs £18. This is £12–13 a month more than fluticasone alone.

Practical advice for prescribing

Salmeterol should not be prescribed as a separate inhaler.
Inhaler technique should be reviewed at every opportunity for all children with asthma.
A valved holding chamber device will improve delivery for most children.

Senna

CLINICAL PHARMACOLOGY

Why and when?	Senna is a **stimulant laxative** used in the **treatment of constipation**, or to clear the bowel in preparation for colonoscopy or surgery. In constipation it should be used in combination with measures to soften stools, such as increasing the amount of high-fibre foods such as fruit, vegetables, bran and high-fibre cereals or encouraging drinking of plenty of water. For constipation, it can be used as maintenance therapy or as **part of a disimpaction regime**n (NICE recommends adding senna if disimpaction is not achieved after 2 weeks of macrogol treatment, or if the macrogol is not tolerated). Senna should be avoided in intestinal obstruction, acute intestinal inflammation (as in IBD), appendicitis and abdominal pain of unknown cause. As it contains lactose it should be avoided in patients on a lactose-free diet.
Absorption	The action of senna **is intra-luminal**, but some (around 5%) is absorbed by the systemic circulation. It is detectable in bile, saliva and the colonic mucosa and breast milk (but is considered safe to use in breastfeeding if the infant is over 1 month).
Biology	Senna is a derivative of the senna plant. The ingested **senna is broken down by the action of colonic bacteria**, the breakdown products directly stimulate increased peristalsis and fluid secretion. Senna can cause stomach cramps from increased peristalsis.
Clearance	Absorbed senna is metabolized by the liver by mechanisms that are not well characterized. There is no recommendation to avoid or adjust dose in hepatic impairment. **Metabolites are excreted in the urine, which may develop a pinkish discolouration**. Most senna is not absorbed and excreted in faeces.

PRACTICAL PRESCRIBING

Dosing	**By mouth** Child 2–3 years: 3.75–15 mg once daily, adjusted to response (2.5–10 mL of 7.5 mg/5 mL syrup) Child 4–5 years: 3.75–30 mg once daily, adjusted to response (2.5–20 mL of 7.5 mg/5 mL syrup) Child 6–17 years: 7.5–30 mg once daily, adjusted to response (5–20 mL of syrup or 1–4 tablets) Tablets are not licensed in children <6 years, syrup is not licensed for children under 2 years.
Administration	Oral preparations are available as tablets, syrup (including sugar-free) or granules. Tablets contain 7.5 mg of senna and syrup contains 7.5 mg/5 mL. Granules also contain the bulking agent ispaghula husk and sugar should be mixed with a drink (at least 150 mL of fluid with a teaspoonful) and swallowed straight away. Alternatively granules can be sprinkled onto food. **A dose (tablets, syrup or granules) should be followed by a full glass of water**. Senna is given once a day; the timing of the dose will not change its effect, but it is worth considering the time it will be convenient to pass stool: **oral preparations produce a bowel movement in 6–12 hours**, rectal preparations generally produce a bowel movement within 2 hours. Giving the dose at the same time of day will incorporate it into the child's routine, which is an important aspect of management of functional constipation. Some recommend giving at night so that the abdominal cramps occur during sleep.
Drug errors and safety	Overdose or prolonged use can result in diarrhoea and water loss, as well as electrolyte disturbance: hypokalaemia, hypernatraemia, hypocalcaemia, hypermagnesaemia and hyperphosphataemia. For this reason senna should be used with caution when used in combination with other drugs that may influence these, or be influenced by these electrolytes (i.e. digoxin). There is a very **small risk** of developing an **atonic** (non-functioning) **colon with prolonged use of stimulant laxatives**. Melanosis coli (reversible pigmentation of the colon seen on colonoscopy) can occur with chronic use, this is asymptomatic and of no consequence. If a dose is missed it should be repeated, but not if the next dose is due in less than 12 hours. If a child vomits within 30 minutes of an oral dose being administered, the dose should be repeated.
Monitoring	The dose of senna should be titrated to response with the **minimum effective dose** being used. Routine monitoring is not required.
Cost	Senna is available over the counter for children aged 12 years and over and prices vary. On prescription senna is **relatively cheap** costing £4.76 for a 500 mL bottle (4–5p per dose) or £2.13 for 100 tablets (2p per dose).

Sodium picosulfate

CLINICAL PHARMACOLOGY

Why and when?	Sodium picosulfate is a **stimulant laxative**, which acts locally in the colon and rectum. It may be used **in conjunction** with osmotic laxatives to treat **constipation**, or it may form the basis of a **colorectal cleansing preparation** to be used prior to diagnostic colonoscopy. It is not often used in isolation to treat constipation, as a better treatment effect is seen when stools are softened with an osmotic laxative first.
Absorption	Sodium picosulfate itself is **not absorbed** from the gastrointestinal tract. It is metabolized by gut bacteria into its active form bis-(p-hydroxyphenyl)-pyridyl-2 methane (BHPM) in the large intestine. Only a small fraction of this is absorbed unchanged.
Biology	Sodium picosulfate itself has no laxative properties and therefore it is a **prodrug**. It is converted into the active laxative compound, BHPM, in the distal segment of the intestine. It is hydrolysed by intestinal brush border enzymes and colonic bacteria. It then stimulates of the mucosa of both the large intestine and of the rectum, resulting in colonic peristalsis. Mucosal stimulation also promotes water and electrolyte accumulation in the bowel, resulting in a degree of stool softening effect as well as stimulation of defecation.
Clearance	Following conversion, minimal amounts of BHPM are absorbed – these are almost completely conjugated in the intestinal wall and the liver to form the inactive BHPM-glucuronide. The majority of this is eliminated mostly via the faeces and biliary tract, although a small amount (approx. 10%) is excreted in urine.

PRACTICAL PRESCRIBING

Dosing	For constipation, sodium picosulfate should be commenced at a dose of **2.5 mg once daily**, this is usually advised to be given at bedtime as the expected onset of action will be 6–12 hours after taking the dose. It can then be **increased in 2.5 mg increments** up to a maximum dose of 10 mg in children under 4 years, or 20 mg for children aged 4 years and over. This dose may continue for a number of days until regular passage of soft stools is achieved, at which time the dose should be gradually reduced and eventually stopped. Prolonged use may lead to electrolyte disturbances.
Side effects and considerations for use	The most common side effects are diarrhoea and abdominal cramps. Less commonly, there may be nausea, vomiting or dizziness. In cases of significant or persistent diarrhoea, or prolonged use of the medication, dehydration or electrolyte disturbances (particularly hyponatraemia and hypokalaemia) can occur. This risk is increased with concomitant use of diuretics or steroids. **Notably, some preparations of sodium picosulfate use ethanol as an excipient; one branded preparation contains 4.8% vol. alcohol.**
Cost	Sodium picosulfate is available as an oral solution (1 mg/mL). All formulations are **relatively cheap**. A 100 mL bottle costs £2.37 and a 300 mL bottle costs £7.10. For a child who begins treatment with a dose of 2.5 mg and increases daily in 2.5 mg increments to an effective dose of 10 mg, which then continues for 5 days, this would be an equivalent cost of £1.54. Sodium picosulfate is also co-formulated with other laxatives (often magnesium oxide) in the form of a powder for reconstitution into an oral solution for use as a bowel cleaning preparation.

Sodium valproate

CLINICAL PHARMACOLOGY

Why and when?	Valproate has a wide spectrum of antiepileptic activity. It is **effective in many kinds of epilepsy**, being particularly useful in certain types of infantile epilepsy, where **its lack of sedative action** is important. It is helpful in adolescents who exhibit both tonic–clonic or myoclonic seizures as well as absence seizures. Valproate is also used in psychiatric conditions such as bipolar depressive illness (as a mood stabilizer) and **sometimes to treat migraine**. Valproate is **highly teratogenic** with harmful neurodevelopmental effects seen in c.30% of pregnancies. It should not be prescribed to women or girls of child-bearing age unless a pregnancy prevention programme is in place and then only if other medications are not effective or tolerated.
Absorption	Sodium valproate is **well absorbed** from the gut (70–100%). In order to reduce gastric upset, conventional formulation tablets should be taken with food. Plasma protein binding of valproate is high (90–95% at low to moderate plasma concentrations) but the proportion of free drug rises with increasing blood concentration. It is **rapidly transported across the blood–brain barrier** via an anion exchange transporter. Slow diffusion into and out of neurons may partly explain why the **drug concentration in plasma does not correlate with its therapeutic effect**.
Biology	Valproate is a simple monocarboxylic acid, chemically unrelated to any other class of antiepileptic drug (AED). **It has multiple actions** but the contribution of each to the known clinical effects is poorly understood. Valproate **potentiates the effect of the inhibitory amino acid γ-aminobutyric acid (GABA)**, possibly by enhanced synthesis and release, and reduced degradation. It also **attenuates the excitatory action of glutamate at N-methyl-D-aspartate (NMDA) receptors** and facilitates **inhibition of voltage-gated T-type Calcium channels**. There is also a **use-dependent blockade of transmembrane Na channels**, thus stabilizing neuronal membranes. The immediate anticonvulsant effects may be due to extracellular actions on neuronal ion channels, but slow diffusion into neurons produces delayed intracellular effects. **The full benefit of treatment may not be apparent for several weeks.**
Clearance	In older children valproate is primarily metabolized in the liver by glucuronidation and is then excreted renally. The sulfation pathway predominates in neonates. It has a relatively long but variable **half-life of 9–21 hours**. Valproate is a non-specific metabolic inhibitor, both of its own metabolism, and that of other anticonvulsants including lamotrigine, phenytoin and carbamazepine. To avoid toxicity, patients taking valproate and starting such drugs as second-line therapy should receive lower doses of the second anticonvulsant. By contrast, the metabolism of valproate is accelerated by enzyme-inducing drugs, e.g. carbamazepine. Sodium valproate should be avoided in those with liver failure and hepatotoxicity. The dose should be reduced in those with renal failure.

PRACTICAL PRESCRIBING

Dosing for oral/ rectal routes	Neonates: 20 mg/kg once daily initially then usual maintenance of 10 mg/kg twice daily.
	Child 1 month–11 years: 10–15 mg/kg daily in 1–2 divided doses (max/dose 600 mg) increasing every 1–2 weeks to a maintenance 25–30 mg/kg daily in 2 divided doses. Doses of up to 60 mg/kg daily in 2 divided doses may be used in some forms of epilepsy under specialist guidance.
	Older child 12–17 years: 600 mg daily in 1–2 divided doses and this is increased in steps of 150–300 mg every 3 days; maintenance 1–2 g daily in 2 divided doses; maximum 2.5 g per day.
Administration	Oral sodium valproate is available as 40 mg/mL suspension, modified-release tablets (200 mg, 300 mg, 500 mg), gastric resistant tablets (200 mg, 500 mg) and 100 mg crushable tablets. Modified-release granules are also available. IV preparations come as powder for reconstitution with 5% glucose or 0.9% sodium chloride solution, to be given over 3–5 minutes. For rectal administration, oral solution may be given rectally. This may require dilution with water to prevent rapid expulsion and should be retained for 15 minutes. If treatment is stopped it should be withdrawn gradually over 1–2 months.
	Bioavailability varies by formulation and care should be taken when switching between different oral formulations. **Children should be maintained on a specific manufacturer's brand or generic product.**
Side effects and considerations for use	Liver dysfunction (including liver failure) can occur. The risk is higher in those <3 years with co-morbidities. It usually occurs in the first 6 months of treatment and those taking multiple AEDs are at higher risk. **Changes in behaviour** may occur and are distressing to families. Children may report hunger or loss of appetite. Some report nausea, abdominal pain, diarrhoea or vomiting. A few notice hair loss. Whilst this usually grows back it may be slightly curlier and darker than before. Uncommon but serious side effects include pancreatitis, pancytopenia or isolated thrombocytopenia. Parents should be warned about the signs of these, and liver failure, so that they present for urgent review.
Monitoring	**Monitoring of blood concentrations is only useful to assess compliance.** It is, however, necessary to check blood indices (full blood counts, liver function, electrolytes) if doses exceed 40 mg/kg daily. Raised liver enzymes are usually transient.
Cost	Whilst valproate is **relatively cheap**, the cost does vary between preparations. Oral suspension (200 mg/5 mL) costs between £5.94 and £9.33 for 300 mL and the IV injection costs £15 per 400 mg ampoule. The cost for 200 mg, 300 mg, 500 mg and 100 mg crushable tablets are around 11p, 17p, 29p and 6p for each tablet. 1g of the modified release granules costs around 41p.

Spironolactone

CLINICAL PHARMACOLOGY

Why and when?	Spironolactone is a **potassium-sparing diuretic**. It is primarily used to treat heart failure and oedematous conditions such as nephrotic syndrome and ascites. Spironolactone induces diuresis concurrently with potassium retention. Therefore, it is often combined with other diuretics (loop diuretics, thiazides) or amphotericin in **order to prevent hypokalaemia**. As a diuretic, it reduces the systemic blood pressure and it is used in the treatment of hypertension. Spironolactone antagonizes the action of aldosterone and it is useful in the management of hyperaldosteronism.
Absorption and distribution	Spironolactone is **well absorbed** from the gastrointestinal tract. The bioavailability improves significantly when it is taken with food and can reach up to 90%. Following absorption spironolactone is highly bound to plasma proteins (>90%).
Biology	Spironolactone is a potassium-sparing diuretic belonging to the class of **aldosterone antagonists**. It binds to the aldosterone intracellular cytoplasmic receptor at the collecting tube of the nephrons. The spironolactone–receptor complex is inactive resulting in a failure to stimulate the Na^+/K^+ exchange sites of the collecting tubule. Thus, it prevents Na^+ reabsorption and, therefore, K^+ and H^+ secretion. Spironolactone also exhibits a **moderate antiandrogen activity by blocking the androgen receptors**. This can result in undesirable side effects.
Clearance	Spironolactone is extensively and rapidly metabolized by the liver and has a **short elimination half-life of 1.4 hours**. The major metabolites of spironolactone are pharmacologically active and have much longer half-lives than the parent drug (around 12–18 hours depending on the metabolite). Thus, spironolactone **exerts its pharmacological action mainly through its metabolites**. The majority of spironolactone is eliminated by the kidneys, while minimal amounts are handled by biliary excretion.

Prescribing medicines with variable concentrations

A few medicines used in paediatric practice are only available as 'special' formulations. These include several potentially toxic drugs and cardiac medications like captopril. When re-prescribed and particularly when completing discharge letters it is very important to stipulate the correct dose (in mg) and concentration (in mg/mL) of the medicine. Whenever possible, do NOT change the concentration as families get very confused and often revert to the previous amount rather than reading the new instructions on the label. Take great care if more than one concentration of a liquid formulation exists.

PRACTICAL PRESCRIBING

Dosing	The dose is dependent on the age of the child, the severity of the oedematous condition and the renal function. The initial recommended daily dose is **1–2 mg/kg for neonates** and **1–3 mg/kg for older children**. Children older than 11 years receive 50–100 mg per day. The total daily dose is given in **1–2 divided doses**. In cases that do not respond to initial doses, the total daily dose can be increased up to 7 mg/kg for neonates and 9 mg/kg for children, but should not exceed 400 mg. In acute renal insufficiency or severe chronic renal impairment, spironolactone should be avoided. No dose adjustment is necessary for hepatic impairment.
Administration	Spironolactone is administered orally and is available as tablets and oral suspension. Tablets are available in strengths of 25 mg, 50 mg and 100 mg each. Oral suspensions are available in various concentrations (5, 10, 25, 50 or 100 mg/mL) from a special manufacturer **and great care must be taken to ensure that the same concentration is prescribed and dispensed** to reduce the risks of a drug error. Doses should also be prescribed in milligrams and not in millilitres to reduce the error risk. Spironolactone should be administered after meals or with small amounts of food to improve absorption.
Side effects and interactions	Spironolactone may cause hyponatraemia, hyperkalaemia, hyperuricaemia and acute renal failure. Hyperkalaemia is a reason to discontinue the medication. As a moderate androgen antagonist, spironolactone has a variety of side effects: alopecia, **gynaecomastia**, benign breast tumour, breast pain, changes in libido, hypertrichosis and menstrual disturbances. Its use has also been associated with agranulocytosis, leukopenia and thrombocytopenia. Hypersensitivity reactions such as Stevens–Johnson syndrome have been described. Other side effects include confusion, dizziness, drowsiness, gastrointestinal disturbances, hepatotoxicity, leg cramps, malaise and rash. The antihypertensive and potassium-sparing effect of spironolactone may be enhanced when it is administered with medications that reduce systemic blood pressure and cause hyperkalaemia.
Monitoring	**Routine monitoring of electrolytes is advised** especially when they are administered in patients with renal impairment. In the occurrence of hyperkalaemia, spironolactone should be discontinued. Care should be taken because of the different strengths of oral solution/suspension available (to be used in an off-label manner), which can increase the risk of medication errors.
Cost	Spironolactone tablets are **cheap** cost for a pack of 28 tablets are £ 0.94 for 25 mg, £4.26 for 50 mg and £1.76 for 100 mg. The cost of oral suspension is much higher and dependent upon the manufacturer.

Surfactant: pulmonary

CLINICAL PHARMACOLOGY

Why and when?	Surfactant is produced within type 2 pneumocytes and is mixture of phospholipids (85%), neutral lipids and specific proteins (10%). The main phospholipid, **dipalmitoyl-phosphatidylcholine** (DPPC), forms a stable monolayer within alveoli. It leads to a reduction in the surface tension and counteracts collapsing forces at end-expiration. Low-molecular-weight surfactant proteins (Sp) Sp-B and Sp-C are essential for structural organization and functional stability. Congenital Sp-B deficiency leads to lethal respiratory failure in the newborn. In comparison, Sp-C deficiency only manifests as interstitial lung disease in later childhood. The other two surfactant proteins, Sp-A and Sp-D, have important immune function mainly in host defence responses to pathogen invasion.
	Its deficiency in newborn infants, both preterm and term, leads to **respiratory distress syndrome** (RDS). Exogenous surfactant is administered intratracheally to treat RDS. Exogenous surfactants are broadly of two categories – natural and synthetic. Natural surfactants are extracted from bovine or porcine lungs and contain Sp-B. Synthetic surfactants licensed for clinical use do not contain Sp-B but newer synthetic surfactants are being developed that contain 'protein analogue'.
Absorption	When given by the intratracheal route, surfactant works almost immediately. Its action is dependent upon it **remaining within the airway**. This results in a rapid reduction in surface tension and significant improvements in oxygenation. Surfactant is then recycled and degraded within the lungs. The individual components probably have different durations of persistence within the airways, with surfactant proteins being cleared more slowly.
Biology	Surfactant is one of the most widely studied pharmaceutical products in neonatal medicine. Recent randomized trials suggest that there may not be any significant advantage in giving prophylactic surfactant therapy after intubation at delivery because of more widespread use of non-invasive mechanical respiratory support, such as nasal continuous distending positive pressure (CPAP). It is a good practice to give the first dose of surfactant at the **earliest opportunity after intubation** in preterm infants under 30 weeks' gestation.
Clearance	The precise **half-life of surfactant depends on many factors** within the lung. It can be inactivated by blood, meconium or inflammatory exudate. This is what informs the dosing and frequency of surfactant therapy in neonates. Larger doses may need to be considered with infection and meconium aspiration. Endogenous surfactant clearance happens through recycling and degradation within the lungs. Its biological half-life is **about 12 hours** but doses may be required more frequently. In clinical practice, it is common to give a second dose of surfactant 4–6 hours after initial dosing if a baby continues to require mechanical ventilation.

PRACTICAL PRESCRIBING

Dosing	Poractant alfa: 100–200 mg/kg (1.25–2.5 mL/kg) intratracheally to treat RDS. Maximum 400 mg/kg per course.
	Additional doses of 100 mg/kg can be given after 4–6 hours, if the baby continues to remain ventilated and requires support with mean airway pressure of >7 cm of water and FiO_2 of >40%, or if there are radiological signs of pneumonia. 100 mg/kg may be considered when using prophylactically.
	Beractant: 100 mg/kg (4 mL/kg) intratracheally in 2–3 aliquots.
	Up to 3 further doses can be given over the next 48 hours, at least 6 h apart.
Administration	Vials are to be stored at 4°C and **used after warming** to room temperature; invert gently without shaking to resuspend active ingredients. Once brought to room temperature vials are not to be returned to the refrigerator more than 8 h later.
	It is standard practice to instill surfactant **through an endotracheal tube using a fine catheter** in a supine ventilated baby after clearing any secretions and pre-oxygenating in order to reduce desaturation and bradycardia episodes subsequently. It can be given **over less than 1 minute** even though manufacturers still recommend giving over 4 min. It is also a good practice to give a few positive pressure breaths after surfactant administration to facilitate uniform distribution within both lungs. Alternative approaches to surfactant administration include using a fine catheter passed through the larynx in unintubated infants or via laryngeal mask. Such approaches are not the standard of care and are still evolving.
Drug errors and safety	Surfactant administration is **generally well tolerated**. Episodes of desaturation and bradycardia can be minimized by pre-oxygenation of the lungs. Respiratory acidosis and pulmonary haemorrhage are described but uncommon. Rapid increase in tidal volume delivery due to improved lung compliance poses a **risk for air leak** (pneumothorax) and can be prevented by appropriate ventilatory weaning.
Monitoring	Infants requiring surfactant therapy will have continuous monitoring of vital parameters, including heart rate, blood pressure, temperature, oxygen saturation as well as intermittent blood gas. Chest X-ray is recommended and may be repeated for clinical indications.
Cost	Surfactants are **relatively expensive treatments**. Poractant alfa is available in vials of 120 mg (1.5 mL) and 240 mg (3 mL) costing £280 and £550, respectively. Beractant is available as a 200 mg (8 mL) vial costing £310.

Tacrolimus

CLINICAL PHARMACOLOGY

Why and when?	As an **immunosuppressive drug**, tacrolimus has multiple indications in children. It is prescribed in **moderate-to-severe eczema** in those over the age of 2 who are unresponsive to conventional treatments. In eczema, it is a short-term treatment with the aim of causing remission from eczema symptoms. It can also be used following solid organ transplants as prophylaxis for graft rejection. This includes liver, kidney and heart transplants. Tacrolimus should be started promptly; within 12–24 hours of transplantation without antibody induction.
Absorption and distribution	When given orally, has a low but variable **bioavailability of approximately 20%**. Plasma concentrations are usually highest 1–3 hours following the dose. When it enters the circulation most tacrolimus is **bound to erythrocytes and plasma proteins**. The volume of distribution in children seems to be higher (almost twice) than that observed in adults. When tacrolimus is applied topically for eczema treatment, systemic bioavailability is extremely low (3–4%) even in children with active eczema who have impaired skin membrane integrity.
Biology	Tacrolimus is a **macrolide calcineurin inhibitor**. It was first isolated from *Streptomyces tsukubaensis*, an actinobacteria found in soil. **Tacrolimus acts on T cells**. Usually, T-cell receptor activation causes an increase in intracellular calcium within the T cell. Following an intracellular signalling cascade calcineurin dephosphorylates the nuclear factor of activated T cells (NFAT). NFAT then increases the activity of genes that transcribe pro-inflammatory cytokines, such as interleukin-2. Tacrolimus **prevents calcineurin dephosphorylating** and therefore reduces the production of pro-inflammatory cytokines and therefore the immune response.
Clearance	Tacrolimus is metabolized by the **cytochrome P450 system** in the liver. This therefore means it has a number of interactions with other materials metabolized by the cytochrome P450 system, including food and drugs. It has a number of inactive metabolites that are usually excreted via faeces. Its elimination half-life is **variable ranging between 3.5 and 40 hours** with an average of 12 hours. The variability in half-life and absorption necessitates drug level monitoring when used for immunosuppression.

PRACTICAL PRESCRIBING

Dosing	Topical for eczema: for a child aged 2–15, a fingertip unit of 0.03% ointment of tacrolimus can be applied twice daily to affected areas, reducing to once daily with improvement. For older children (16–17) 0.1% ointment can be applied twice daily, and this is reduced to once daily or 0.03% ointment with improvement of the lesions. If no improvement is seen after 2 weeks, it should be discontinued.
	There are 3 different oral preparations of tacrolimus. **Switching between different oral formulations** is **not recommended** and requires careful therapeutic monitoring and should only be done under close supervision of a transplant specialist. Doses of tacrolimus are brand- and transplant-dependent.
	In general, children require higher doses per kilogram of bodyweight than adults. Typical oral maintenance doses for children are 300 micrograms (mcg)/kg daily in 2 divided doses but may be lower in individuals who have had antibody induction prior to heart transplantation.
Administration	Tacrolimus can be given orally, topically or intravenously. Both tablets and an oral suspension of tacrolimus are available; the oral suspension is much more expensive. Granules to prepare an oral solution are also available.
Drug errors and safety	As an immunosuppressive drug, tacrolimus increases risk of infection. It can also cause nephropathy, cardiomyopathy in children and pancytopenia. It can prolong the QT interval. Regular ECGs are required during childhood to **screen for cardiomyopathy**. Long-term immunosuppression increases the risk of skin cancers and therefore high factor sunscreen should be used. **Switching between brands is associated with toxicity and graft rejection**.
Monitoring	With systemic use, **regular tacrolimus peak and trough blood concentration levels should be taken**. Typically this will be weekly initially and increase to monthly and less often if stable. Assays for tacrolimus levels differ between hospitals, and local guidelines should be followed to ensure adequacy of dose. If doses have been missed or may be ineffective (for example following vomiting), trough levels should be taken to ensure the tacrolimus levels are correct.
Cost	Tacrolimus is a **relatively expensive drug**. 500 mcg tacrolimus capsules costs almost £1 each. Granules are more expensive still, costing about £7/g. A single 5 mg/1 mL ampoule for IV infusion costs almost £60. Topical tacrolimus ointment costs £20–25 for 30 g of 0.03% preparation.

Tobramycin

CLINICAL PHARMACOLOGY

Why and when?	Tobramycin is an **aminoglycoside antibiotic** with a wide spectrum of antibacterial activity. It is effective against ***Pseudomonas aeruginosa*** (PA) and is therefore commonly used in children with **cystic fibrosis** (CF). Intravenous (IV) tobramycin is used alongside another IV anti-PA antibiotic, such as ceftazidime, to treat pulmonary exacerbations caused by PA. Inhaled tobramycin can be prescribed as a single 28-day course to eradicate new isolates of PA or on alternate months to improve lung function and reduce pulmonary exacerbations in those with chronic PA infection.
Absorption and distribution	Aminoglycosides are poorly absorbed from the gastrointestinal tract. After parenteral administration, aminoglycosides are primarily distributed within the extracellular fluid.
Biology	Tobramycin has bacteriostatic and bactericidal actions. Irreversible **binding to the 30S bacterial ribosome** and inhibition of bacterial protein synthesis makes it bacteriostatic. Tobramycin is bactericidal as it creates a fissure in the bacteria outer cell membrane leading to leakage of intracellular contents and enhanced antibiotic uptake. The bactericidal effects are concentration-dependent with a peak concentration (C_{max})/minimum inhibitory concentration (MIC) ratio >10 being a marker of therapeutic response
Clearance	There is no protein binding of tobramycin and it is cleared almost entirely by glomerular filtration. The **plasma elimination half-life is 2–3 hours** although longer in infants (especially if low birth weight) and in those with impaired renal function.
Administration	**Once and three times daily tobramycin are equally effective in treating CF pulmonary exacerbations in children but once daily is preferred due to evidence of less nephrotoxicity and convenience.** For IV infusion tobramycin is diluted with glucose 5% or sodium chloride 0.9% and given over 20–60 minutes.

In obese patients it is recommended that ideal weight for height is used to calculate the parenteral dose. This reduces the risk of overdosage and toxicity (see Side effects below).

PRACTICAL PRESCRIBING

Dosing	In children without CF, where tobramycin is used to treat possible PA infections (including meningitis) initial doses are somewhat lower (4–5 mg/kg in neonates given every 36 hours for babies <32 weeks and every 24 hours for those over 32 weeks and 7 mg/kg once daily in other age groups).
	Typical doses in children with CF are:
	IV tobramycin infusion: **10 mg/kg (maximum 660 mg) once daily,** then adjusted according to serum concentrations.
	Inhalation of nebulized tobramycin (Bramitob® or Tobi®): 300 mg twice daily.
	Inhalation of dry powder tobramycin (Tobi®): 112 mg twice daily.
Side effects	Tobramycin is nephrotoxic, ototoxic and vestibulotoxic. Many of the effects are cumulative and for children with CF these represent important long-term sequelae of treatment.
	Nephrotoxicity: use of IV tobramycin is associated with **acute kidney injury** (AKI) and repeated courses can cause subclinical kidney damage leading to chronic kidney disease (CKD). Tobramycin is nephrotoxic as after glomerular filtration, 5–15% of the dose is retained in the proximal tubules.
	Ototoxicity: **permanent hearing loss** is a recognized side effect of tobramycin. Two mutations affecting the mitochondrial 12S ribosomal RNA gene predispose carriers to tobramycin ototoxicity.
	Vestibulotoxicity: **this can occur independently** from ototoxicity and causes symptoms of dizziness and feeling light-headed. It results from tobramycin damaging the hair cells in the vestibular system. Symptoms can slowly improve when treatment is stopped but can also be permanent.
Monitoring	IV tobramycin has a **narrow therapeutic range** and monitoring of plasma concentration is required to reduce the side effects. In once-daily dosing, the pre-dose concentration should be <1 mg/L. If it is higher than this, the time between doses should be increased to 36 or 48 hours. Post dose levels are only required if using multiple daily dose regimen.
Cost	Tobramycin is a **fairly expensive antibiotic**. A 2-week course of IV tobramycin for a 24-kg child costs approximately £650. 1 month's supply of nebulized tobramycin costs approximately £1200. 1 month's supply of dry powder tobramycin cost approximately £1800.

Tranexamic acid

CLINICAL PHARMACOLOGY

Why and when?	Tranexamic acid is an **antifibrinolytic drug** used to medically manage excessive bleeding and related coagulopathy. It is considered most valuable in **controlling haemorrhage** – commonly this is in the context of paediatric trauma and surgery. In theatre, the National Institute for Health and Care Excellence (NICE) guidance suggests tranexamic acid prophylaxis should be considered for any surgery where blood loss is expected to exceed 10% of blood volume. Whilst major and refractory bleeding are clear indications for the use of tranexamic acid, it is commonly prescribed to treat and prevent bleeding in children with **menorrhagia and haemophilia**. In all cases, the principal aim is to reduce blood loss and transfusion rates. Beyond bleeding, tranexamic acid can also be used for the prevention of acute attacks of hereditary angioedema or chronic spontaneous urticaria/angioedema unresponsive to antihistamines.
Absorption	Pharmacokinetic data on tranexamic acid are almost exclusively derived from adult studies. Administered orally, gastrointestinal absorption of tranexamic acid delivers 30–50% of the given dose and this is unaffected by food intake. Intravenously, peak plasma concentrations are rapidly achieved. At therapeutic plasma levels the protein bound proportion of the drug is 3%. Tranexamic acid does not bind to albumin, instead binding exclusively to circulating plasminogen. It is hydrophilic and patients with increased total body water (e.g. neonates) are thought to need higher doses.
Biology	Tranexamic acid **blocks normal fibrinolytic responses**. As a synthetic lysine analogue, it reversibly blocks the lysine binding sites on plasminogen and prevents its conversion to plasmin. At higher concentrations **plasmin itself is directly inhibited**. This results in the systemic preservation of fibrin clots, circulating fibrinogen and procoagulant factors V and VIII. Through the same mechanism, it is thought that the inflammatory cascades mediated by plasmin are also inhibited by tranexamic acid, supporting its efficacy in the treatment of menorrhagia. Though the mechanism is undetermined, the role of tranexamic acid in the management of hereditary angioedema and chronic spontaneous urticaria/angioedema are linked to a **reduction in bradykinin** caused by its downregulation of factor XII. It has a plasma **half life of approximately 3 hours**.
Clearance	Tranexamic acid is cleared renally after minimal metabolism. More than 95% of the drug is excreted in urine unchanged. After 24 hours, urinary excretion of a 10–15 mg/kg dose is 90% for intravenous (IV) administration. Dose reduction and careful monitoring are recommended in children with even mild renal impairment due to the risks of accumulation.

PRACTICAL PRESCRIBING

Dosing	Dosage and administration protocols vary significantly across UK paediatric centres. Age and body weight should be considered and caution exercised when prescribing for neonates, infants and renally impaired children. For the acute inhibition of fibrinolysis a **10 mg/kg IV bolus, given 2–3 times a day (max. 1 g per dose), is recommended**. The therapeutic levels can be maintained by use of a continuous infusion at a rate of 45 mg/kg/24 hours. When used orally for acute episodes of angioedema, haemophilia bleeding prophylaxis or as a second-line treatment for chronic urticarial/ angioedema 15–25 mg/kg (maximum 1.5 g) 2–3 times per day is recommended. In haemophilia the prophylactic dose should be given preoperatively. For menorrhagia, young women over 12 years should be prescribed 1 g three times a day (not exceeding 4 g per day) for up to 4 days from the first day of menstruation.
Administration	Rapid infusion may cause dizziness and hypotension and bolus injections **should be administered slowly over a period of 10 minutes** to reduce this. For infusion, tranexamic acid can be diluted with a number of different solutions including NaCl (sodium chloride) 0.9% or glucose 5%. Administration of tranexamic acid to children under the age of 1 (or any age as a continuous infusion) is unlicensed, as is its use for reduction of blood loss in cardiac surgery.
Drug errors and safety	A large range of doses (up to 100 mg/kg) have been reported in major trauma with few reported adverse effects; signs of toxicity and overdose include nausea, vomiting, hypotension, malaise and convulsions. Management of overdose is supportive. In children under the age of 2 (or with renal impairment) the drug should prescribed with caution and only when benefits outweigh the risks. It is **contraindicated in severe renal impairment** and should not be given if disseminated intravascular coagulation (DIC) is suspected or diagnosed. For longer-term use, care should be taken when co-prescribing with other pro-thrombotic drugs (most commonly oral contraceptives).
Monitoring	Long-term use in hereditary angioedema warrants regular liver function testing.
Cost	Tranexamic acid is a **relatively cheap** medicine. In secondary care, ampoules of tranexamic acid for injection cost around £1.50 each; an ampoule contains 500 mg/5 mL solution. In tablet form, 500 mg of tranexamic acid costs approximately 0.25p per tablet.

Trimethoprim

CLINICAL PHARMACOLOGY

Why and when?	Trimethoprim is an **antibiotic** that can only be given orally, as a tablet or suspension. It is mainly used for the **treatment** or **prophylaxis** of **urinary tract infections** (UTIs), but can be used in treatment or prevention of respiratory tract infections (RTIs).
	Trimethoprim is sometimes combined with sulfamethoxazole, another folate antagonist, as the two antibiotics work synergistically. This combination is called **co-trimoxazole** and can be given orally or intravenously. Its main use is the treatment or prophylaxis of (*Pneumocystis jirovecii (carinii)*) infections, but it is emerging as an option in other infections due to growing antibiotic resistance.
Absorption	Oral trimethoprim has a **high bioavailability** of close to 100%, and therefore is suitable to be given by the oral route. It is advised to be given or taken on an empty stomach. Trimethoprim reaches peak concentrations in the blood about 1–4 hours after ingestion. The drug has a wide distribution with roughly 45% being bound to plasma proteins.
Biology	Its mechanism of action is **inhibiting** the enzyme **dihydrofolate reductase (DHFR)**, which produces tetrahydrofolate. This molecule is needed in the synthesis of a number of amino acids, and also the synthesis of deoxyribonucleic acid (DNA). Trimethoprim is a **bacteriostatic drug**, which is active against a number of organisms, including *Escherichia coli*, *Pneumocystis jirovecii*, *Proteus* and *Klebsiella* species.
	Trimethoprim resistance has been rapidly rising. A third of organisms isolated from UTI samples analyzed in labs across the NHS in 2016 were found to be resistant to the drug. Resistance may be due to several mechanisms, including increased production of DHFR by organisms, plasmid-mediated changes in DHFR causing it to be resistant to inhibition by trimethoprim and changes in cell permeability causing reduction of drug uptake by bacteria.
Clearance	Less than 20% of trimethoprim is metabolized in the liver. Most of each dose is excreted **renally** via filtration and secretion. Its **half-life is about 10–16 hours**.
	It is recommended that prescribers use half the normal dose from day 1 if the creatinine clearance is <15 mL/min, and using half the normal dose after day 3 if the creatinine clearance is 15–30 mL/min.

PRACTICAL PRESCRIBING

Dosing	**Age-** and **weight**-banded dosing regimens exist. The treatment dose is usually **4 mg/kg twice daily** (after the age of 4 weeks), for treatment of UTIs/RTIs, up to a maximum of 400 mg daily.

A dose of **1–2 mg/kg once daily** is used for prophylaxis of UTIs, up to a maximum of 100 mg daily.

A dose of 5 mg/kg 6–8-hourly can be used for the treatment of mild to moderate *Pneumocystis jirovecii* infections in conjunction with dapsone in patients who cannot tolerate co-trimoxazole. |
| Administration | Oral trimethoprim is available in 100 mg or 200 mg **tablets**, or in a 50 mg/5 mL **suspension**, which can be sugar-free. |
| Drug errors and safety | Trimethoprim should not be used in patients who have a known **folate deficiency** due to its mechanism of action. Caution should be taken in neonates and patients with acute porphyrias. The most common side effects are **headaches**, skin **rashes**, **nausea**, **vomiting** and **diarrhoea**.

More serious side effects are **hyperkalaemia**, due to antagonism of the epithelial sodium channel of the distal tubule, **elevated creatinine** concentrations as trimethoprim competes with creatinine for secretion into the renal tubule, and **megaloblastic anaemia** due to reduced folate levels. Renal failure and hyperkalaemia are more commonly seen in the elderly population treated with trimethoprim for UTIs when compared with other antibiotics. |
| Monitoring | Routine monitoring is not required but a **reduced dose** is needed if a child has **poor renal function.** If a child is on long-term trimethoprim therapy, then a 3–6-monthly full blood count is advisable. |
| Cost | Trimethoprim is **inexpensive**. Prices vary between manufacturers but currently it costs between 3p and 36p per 100 mg tablet, and between 17p and 54p for the equivalent of 100 mg as oral suspension. |

Vitamin D

CLINICAL PHARMACOLOGY

Why and when?	Vitamin D is **essential for the absorption and utilization of calcium** and **phosphorus**. It maintains neuromuscular and immune functioning. **Prolonged deficiency** of vitamin D during periods of bone growth in children leads to a failure or delay of endochondral calcification at the growth plates of the long bones, which results in **rickets** and an accumulation of excess unmineralized osteoid (bone matrix) in all bones; the low mineral to bone matrix ratio in bone results in osteomalacia.
	The most at risk are those with increased need (babies, adolescents and obese individuals), those with reduced ultraviolet-B (UVB) radiation exposure and with diets low in vitamin D. The term 'vitamin D' embraces a range of compounds including **ergocalciferol** (calciferol, vitamin D_2-plant product), **colecalciferol** (vitamin D_3 – mammal, fish products), **alfacalcidol** (1α-hydroxycholecalciferol) and **calcitriol** (1,25-dihydroxycholecalciferol).
	Most vitamin D supplements require **hydroxylation**, by the kidney and liver, to produce the biologically active form, 1,25-dihydroxycholecalciferol.
Absorption	Under normal circumstances most (c.90%) vitamin D is synthesized following exposure of the skin to UVB radiation. Oral supplementation may be required for those who have become deficient or who cannot gain sufficient natural exposure to UVB wavelength light.
	Oral preparations of vitamin D **are fat-soluble**. Their absorption is limited in any children with fat malabsorption, e.g. cystic fibrosis. A few foods are fortified with small amounts of vitamin D (margarine, infant formula milk, some breakfast cereals) and small amounts are present in red meat and egg yolks (c.30 units vitamin D). Breast milk contains small amounts of vitamin D and these levels are even lower in deficient mothers.
Biology	Vitamin D is converted enzymatically in the **liver to 25-hydroxy-vitamin D** (25[OH]D), the major circulating form of vitamin D, and then in the **kidney to 1,25-dihydroxyvitamin D**, the active form of vitamin D. Levels of 1,25-dihydroxyvitamin D are typically 1000-fold lower than the 25-hydroxy form.
Clearance	The plasma half-life of vitamin D is about **4–6 hours**, although the biological half-life is much longer. It distributes widely into tissues and in particular will be stored in body fat, which may act as both a sink and source for vitamin D. Degradation of vitamin D_2 and D_3 is catalyzed by the 24-hydroxylase enzyme CYP24 (produced in the kidney), which produces inactive water-soluble compounds, which are excreted in bile.

PRACTICAL PRESCRIBING

Dosing	Vitamin D deficiency is defined as a blood level of 25-hydroxy-vitamin D below 25 nmol/L and 'insufficiency' as between 25 and 50 nmol/L. To prevent deficiency, a daily dose of **400 IU** of **colecalciferol** (10 micrograms) is recommended for children.

Deficiency requires treatment for 4-8 weeks. The treatment of symptomatic deficiency is a course of 4-8 weeks with 1000–3000 IU daily for babies up to a year, 3000–6000 IU daily for children up to 12 years of age and 6000–10,000 IU daily for those >12 years. If adherence is likely to be an issue, then higher doses can be given less frequently (i.e. weekly or monthly). |
| Administration | Vitamin D is available as liquid, tablets, chewable tablets or capsules of varying strengths. Combined calcium and vitamin D tablets are available but unless the patient has insufficient calcium intake it is often better, and cheaper, to prescribe a pure vitamin D product. |
| Drug errors, safety and monitoring | Under most circumstances, vitamin D is a safe medicine. Endogenous production of vitamin D following UVB exposure, i.e. 60 minutes of midday summer sun exposure can exceed 10,000 IU in healthy adults. Nonetheless, it is important to assess the clinical response and repeat serum calcium, phosphate and vitamin D levels when on treatment. For children with **rickets or hypocalcaemia** then it is also necessary to monitor blood parathyroid hormone levels and alkaline phosphatase. **Initial blood tests should be weekly**.

Symptoms of acute intoxication can be due to **hypercalcaemia** and include confusion, polyuria, polydipsia, anorexia, vomiting and muscle weakness. Long-term intoxication can cause bone demineralization and pain. |
| Cost | Vitamin D preparations are **relatively cheap**. Tablet forms are the cheapest and a single 1000 IU tablet may cost as little as 1p. Chewable tablets are also available and still fairly cheap, costing about 3p for 400 IU tablets and 7p for 1000 IU tablets. Oral suspension is a little more expensive: 1 mL of 400 IU/1 mL colecalciferol costs c.8p.

Whilst individual prescriptions are inexpensive, collectively spending on vitamin D preparations has **increased dramatically** in recent years in the UK as awareness about deficiency has increased. Annual costs increased from £1647 per 100,000 individuals in 2008 to £28,913 per 100,000 individuals in 2014. |

Vitamin K (Phytomenadione)

CLINICAL PHARMACOLOGY

Why and when?

Vitamin K received its name in 1935, after being known as 'Koagulations vitamin' in German, which means 'clotting vitamin'. It is a fat-soluble vitamin that is mostly acquired from dietary sources, as vitamin K_1 (phylloquinone), and from endogenous sources, by colonic bacterial synthesis, as menaquinones K_2. In children, vitamin K is commonly used in **prophylaxis and treatment of vitamin K deficiency bleeding** (formerly known as haemorrhagic disease of the newborn), and in **coagulopathy** secondary to **impaired absorption or synthesis of vitamin K,** such as obstructive jaundice, coeliac disease, cystic fibrosis and intestinal resection.

Absorption

Whilst **highly variable** between individuals, the systemic availability following an oral dose of vitamin K is approximately 50%. Increased concentrations of blood-coagulation factors are seen within 6–12 hours of an oral dose. Vitamin K is a 'fat-soluble' vitamin. Intestinal absorption follows a well-established pathway that applies to most dietary lipids, which includes bile salt- and pancreatic-dependent solubilization, uptake into the enterocytes of the jejunum and ileum, and their exocytosis as chylomicrons enter the lymphatic system and then the blood via the thoracic duct. The absence or **insufficiency of pancreatic enzymes and bile salts** significantly **impairs the absorption** of vitamin K. Parenteral vitamin K is needed in those with hepatic dysfunction or hepatobiliary obstructive disease.

Biology

Vitamin K is an essential element in the coagulation pathway; it plays a role in activation of vitamin K dependent factors. With the exception of newborns and infants, deficiency is rare. Vitamin K is **not readily transferred through the placenta** to the fetus, and its **excretion in breast milk is poor**. The highest risk period for vitamin K deficiency bleeding is at 3–8 weeks of age. Vitamin K is added to infant formula, therefore exclusively breastfed babies are at highest risk. **Oral prophylaxis** is not effective in patients with underlying cholestatic liver disease and malabsorption.

Individuals with liver disease or malabsorption develop signs of vitamin K deficiency if not replaced or treated. Deficiency of vitamin K means that the carboxylation reaction of the procoagulant factors II, VII, IX, and X cannot proceed. This leads to a **high prothrombin time (PT)**, and there may be bruising, gastrointestinal, genitourinary or cerebral bleeding.

Clearance

Vitamin K metabolism is **relatively rapid** when compared with other fat-soluble vitamins. It proceeds in the liver, via shortening and then conjugation. The cytochrome P450 enzyme group are important in metabolism. Conjugated metabolites are excreted in the urine and bile. In comparison with other fat-soluble vitamins, phylloquinone is poorly retained in the body. Studies with radiolabelled vitamin K indicate that 60–70% is excreted within 5 days.

PRACTICAL PRESCRIBING

Dosing	**Prevention of vitamin K deficiency bleeding:**
	400 microgram (mcg)/kg (max. dose 1 mg) intramuscularly (IM; the most clinically and cost-effective method) or by mouth.
	When the 2 mg dose is given **orally** at birth a **repeated dose is required at 4–7 days,** and in exclusively breastfed infants either a further single 2 mg dose at 1 month of age or a dose of 1–2 mg once-weekly for 12 weeks. **There is a risk that these doses may be forgotten** or fail to be prescribed on discharge from hospital after birth.
	Treatment dosage for vitamin K deficiency bleeding:
	1 mg intravenous (IV)/IM in neonates and 1–3 mg IV/IM in infants.
	Further doses are usually required (up to 8-hourly) depending on coagulation status. It is recommended that vitamin K be given IV and not IM until coagulation normalizes. Serious bleeding, particularly in premature infants or those with liver disease, may require a transfusion of fresh-frozen plasma or whole blood. For bleeding and hypoprothrombinaemia caused by vitamin K deficiency or warfarin therapy in children, a dose of 250–300 mcg/kg is indicated (10 mg maximum).
Side effects and considerations	Vitamin K can be prescribed via orally, IM and IV routes. Konakion® MM Paediatric can be given by all of these routes. Special-order manufacturers include capsule, oral suspension and oral solution.
	There are very few side effects of vitamin K, except the temporary pain of an injection and bruising at the injection site. IV treatment can rarely lead to adverse reactions especially when administered in high doses, the most notable of which is kernicterus. Lower initial doses may be required in jaundiced infants, but risks of bleeding must be balanced against risk of kernicterus.
Monitoring	Blood monitoring is not usually undertaken **unless there is significant bleeding or known high risk of haemorrhage**. PT indicates vitamin K status and response to treatment in deficient cases. PT is more sensitive than activated partial thromboplastin time (APTT). In general, response to administration will cause a shortening of the PT time within few hours. If shortening of the PT is not seen, other coagulation factor deficiencies should be considered.
Cost	Vitamin K **is cheap**. A single 2 mg dose of Konakion MM Paediatric currently costs less than £1 in the UK.

Warfarin

CLINICAL PHARMACOLOGY

Why and when?	Warfarin is an **antithrombotic agent** used in the **treatment and prophylaxis of thrombotic episodes**. When being used for acute treatment of a thrombus it is usually initiated alongside another anticoagulant such as heparin or low-molecular-weight heparin as it takes 3–4 days to take full effect. **Frequent blood tests** to monitor the International Normalized Ratio (INR) **are required** as it has a narrow therapeutic window. It is not licensed for use in children but is still the oral anticoagulant of choice for the treatment of thromboembolism, because of familiarity and the lack of an alternative.
Absorption and distribution	Warfarin is given orally. It is available in tablets or an oral suspension. It has a **bioavailability of almost 100%** unless there is diarrhoea or vomiting. It reaches its peak concentration within 4 hours. It extensively binds to plasma proteins (c.99%) and has a small volume of distribution.
Biology	Warfarin belongs to the drug class '**vitamin K antagonists**'. Vitamin K is an essential co-factor for the synthesis of clotting factors II, VII, IX and X. It promotes the synthesis of γ-carboxyglutamic acid residues in these clotting factors, which is essential for their biological activity. Warfarin inhibits the regeneration of vitamin K_1 epoxide inhibiting the cyclic conversion of vitamin K. This **reduces** the active form of clotting factors **II, VII, IX** and **X by c.30–50%** at therapeutic doses.
Clearance	Warfarin is mostly metabolized in the liver by the cytochrome P450 (CYP) enzymes, predominantly the **CYP2C9 isoenzyme**. The metabolites have very little anticoagulant activity and are mainly excreted into the urine (>90%) with a small amount excreted in bile. The half-life of warfarin is approximately 40 hours but can vary between 20 and 60 hours. CYP2CP is expressed from early life and **children <1 year take slightly longer to achieve therapeutic anticoagulation.** Induction or inhibition of the CYP P450 cytochromes affects warfarin plasma concentrations. Polymorphisms in *CYP2C9* and *VKORC1* affect dosing requirements, but testing for these is not yet established in clinical practice.
Dosing	The dose of warfarin given is very dependent on the INR result. When initiated, the standard dose is 200 micrograms (mcg)/kg (max 10 mg) for one dose followed by 100 mcg/kg (max 5 mg) once daily for the next 3 days. Subsequent doses are then adjusted according to the INR but the usual maintenance dose is between 100 mcg/kg and 300 mcg/kg once daily. Local protocols should be followed and the **INR should always be checked at times of illness** so dose adjusts can take place when needed.
	Formula-fed infants may require higher doses due to vitamin K supplementation in the formula. In contrast, breastfed infants are likely to be more sensitive to warfarin due to low concentrations of vitamin K in breast milk.

PRACTICAL PRESCRIBING

Administration	Warfarin is given orally, either by tablet (available as 0.5 mg, 1 mg, 3 mg or 5 mg) or oral suspension (1 mg/mL). The suspension should be shaken thoroughly before administration. **It is usually taken at the same time every evening** with the standard time recommended as 6pm.
Side effects and interactions	The main adverse consequence of warfarin therapy is **haemorrhage**. Risk factors include those with haematological disorders where bleeding risk is already increased, a history of gastrointestinal bleeding, recent stroke or surgery, uncontrolled hypertension and hyper/hypothyroidism. Other serious side effects include calciphylaxis (vascular calcification with cutaneous necrosis). It presents as a painful rash and is most commonly observed in patients with end-stage renal disease.
	Warfarin interacts with many drugs and a suitable reference should be consulted before prescribing other drugs. Interactions include synergistic effects with **drugs that act on the clotting cascade**; drugs that cause **CYP2CP induction or inhibition**; **antibiotics** that change the gut flora and alter vitamin K absorption; other highly protein-bound drugs may displace warfarin leading to more free, and therefore active, drug in the plasma. **Foodstuffs can also interact with warfarin**. Cranberry and pomegranate have been shown to increase its anticoagulant effect. Foods that contain lots of vitamin K (fortified milks, broccoli, Brussel sprouts and green leafy vegetables) reduce its coagulant effect.
	In overdose, if life-threatening haemorrhage is present, then warfarin must be stopped and a prothrombin complex concentrate given. This should be discussed with the local haematologist or a poisons information service. In non-life-threatening haemorrhage, where anticoagulation can be stopped, phytomenadione (vitamin K) can be given and the INR monitored.
Monitoring	The **dose of warfarin is determined by the INR** and therefore **monitoring is vital** in its use. A baseline prothrombin time should be determined before the initial dose is given. The INR is initially monitored every 24–48 hours and then at longer intervals up to a maximum of every 12 weeks as the patient becomes established on treatment. Any change in the patient's clinical condition, such as intercurrent illness or drug administration, requires more frequent testing. Once the patient is established on treatment, point of care testing using a 'finger prick test' may be more convenient and less traumatic.
	All patients (or carers) should be given an **anticoagulant treatment booklet**. These booklets contain advice on anticoagulant treatment, an alert card to be carried by the patient at all times and a section for recording INR results and dosage information.
Cost	**Tablets are cheap** but **oral solution is fairly expensive**. Warfarin oral solution (1 mg/mL) costs £108 for a 150 mL bottle. By contrast tablets cost between 2p and 4p each.

Appendix 1

Comparison of the different generations of cephalosporins commonly used in children

Generation	Examples	Route	Properties
First	Cefalexin Cefadroxil Cefradine	Oral Oral Oral	Narrower spectrum of activity, mostly Gram-positive activity only. Useful for urinary tract infections (UTIs) and some respiratory tract infections. Cefadroxil has poor activity against *Haemophilus influenzae*. Limited central nervous system (CNS) penetration.
Second	Cefaclor Cefuroxime	Oral Oral/IV	Good activity against *Haemophilus influenzae*. Cefuroxime has better activity against Gram-positive bacteria (e.g. *S. aureus*), especially at higher doses, than third-generation cephalosporins.
Third	Cefixime Cefotaxime Ceftriaxone Ceftazidime	Oral IV/IM IV/IM IV	Cefixime has a long duration of action and the oral solution is particularly palatable. Cefotaxime and ceftriaxone are useful as empiric treatment in sepsis. Ceftazidime has good activity against *Pseudomonas sp*.

Appendix 2

DOSE AND FREQUENCY OF OMALIZUMAB FOR CHILDREN WITH SEVERE PERSISTENT ALLERGIC ASTHMA

Baseline IgE IU/mL	Body weight									
	20-25	>25-30	>30-40	>40-50	>50-60	>60-70	>70-80	>80-90	>90-125	>125-150
≥30-100	75	75	75	150	150	150	150	150	300	300
>100-200	150	150	150	300	300	300	300	300	225	300
>200-300	150	150	225	300	300	225	225	225	300	375
>300-400	225	225	300	225	225	225	300	300	450	525
>400-500	225	300	225	225	300	300	375	375	525	600
>500-600	300	300	225	300	300	375	375	450	600	
>600-700	300	225	300	300	375	450	525	525		
>700-800	225	225	300	375	450	450	525	600		
>800-900	225	225	300	375	450	525	600			
>900-1000	225	300	375	450	525	600				
>1000-1100	300	300	375	450	600					
>1100-1200	300	300	450	525	600					
>1200-1300	300	375	450	525						
>1300-1500	300	375	525	600						

Do not administer

Legend:
- treatment every 4 weeks
- could be switched to q4wk
- mg/kg dose too high to switch
- Too many injections to switch

Appendix 3

	Gluco-corticoid effect*	Mineralo-corticoid effect*	Plasma half-life (hours)	Biological half-life (hours)
Hydrocortisone	1	1	2	8–12
Prednisolone	4	0.8	3–4	12–36
Methylprednisolone	5	0.5	3	12–36
Dexamethasone	30	0	3–4	36–54
Fludrocortisone	15	150	4	24–36

*Potency relative to hydrocortisone

Index

207

Index